Biomechanics and Medicine in Swimming VII

Biomechanics and Medicine in Swimming VII

Edited by
J.P. TROUP, A.P. HOLLANDER,
D. STRASSE, S.W. TRAPPE,
J.M. CAPPAERT and T.A. TRAPPE

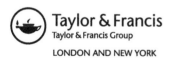

Taylor & Francis
Taylor & Francis Group

LONDON AND NEW YORK

Published by Taylor & Francis
2 Park Square, Milton Park, Abingdon, Oxon, OX14 4RN
711 Third Avenue, New York, NY 10017, USA

Routledge is an imprint of the Taylor & Francis Group, an informa business

First edition 1996

First issued in paperback 2011

© 1996 Taylor & Francis

ISBN 978-0-419-20480-0 (hbk)
ISBN 978-0-415-51439-2 (pbk)

A catalogue record for this book is available from the British Library

Library of Congress Catalog Card Number: 96–69459

Publishers Note
This book has been produced from camera ready copy provided by the individual
contributors.

The publisher has gone to great lengths to ensure the quality of this reprint but
points out that some imperfections in the original may be apparent

Contents

Preface

Swimming faster is the objective of every applied sport scientist and the ultimate target of the investigator's research. While research findings in and of themselves can not result in faster swimming, the interpretation of the results however, can help the practitioner understand how fast swimming will happen. The opportunity to interpret these results takes place at International Meetings as investigators from around the world come together for the sole purpose of discussing and debating how individual study result can contribute to our overall knowledge of faster swimming. In this edition, we have selected the most practical and thought provoking papers from over 80 studies presented at the VIIth Biomechanics and Medicine in Swimming World Congress.

Although these papers can not convey the enthusiastic discussions that took place during the conference, the editors would encourage the reader to take these findings and host your own discussions with colleagues at home. Hopefully, your discussions will lead to additional questions, additional study and new information in all of our quests to better understand how to swim faster.

Finally, special thanks must be given to key people that made the conference organization possible including Cindy Hayes, Conference Secretariat, Carol Zaleski, President of United States Swimming, Ray Essick, Executive Director of United States Swimming, Jan Clarys and Peter Hollander for ISB and Swimming Subcommittee support.

To those who were not able to join us at this conference, it is our hope that reading this proceedings will stimulate you to participate in future swimming conferences.

John P. Troup, Ph.D.
Mystic, Connecticut USA
1995

Foreword

THE HISTORICAL PERSPECTIVE OF SWIMMING SCIENCE

J.P. CLARYS

Experimental Anatomy, Vrije Universiteit Brussels, Belgium

"...Only a part of what was observed in the past was remembered by those who observed it ;.. only a part of what was recorded has survived. ;.. only a part of what has survived has come to the peoples attention ;... only a part of what has come to their attention is credible ;... only a part of what is credible has been grasped ; ... and only part of what has been grasped can be expounded or narrated".

This "reality of the historian" in combination with climatological and geographical differences amongst civilisations, the little practical use of swimming and the individual interpretation of visual historical remainders make it very difficult to tell "the" correct story. Nevertheless it is assumed in riverside cultures that swimming became part of life out of (i) necessity for finding and picking up food (Fig. 1) because of (ii) military reasons e.g. crossing rivers (Fig. 2) due to (iii) religion and self protecting (life saving) influence (Fig. 3) - e.g. the spirit of the death will not find rest if the body was drowned ; and surely out of (iiii) recreational and/or status reasons (Fig. 4) (1) (2) (3) (4) (5).

We are interested in swimming out of other perspectives. We want to look at movement and at performance. We want to appreciate the kinesiology. Observing the two oldest remainders representing swimming (Fig. 5 and 6) and looking at the best known hieroglyphic illustration of a swiming man (or woman)... "the NEBU" (Fig. 7), we do recognize a kind of double backstroke, breastroke (Fig. 5), side stroke or frontcrawl (Fig. 6 and 7). Amazing because we are 5000 and 2100 years BC, (6) (2) (7) and these illustrations are made with a "movement analyses" spirit.

The culturo-historical road to swimming science is long, very long, but the start may be assumed in the field of swimming medicine. We already appreciated a "kind of" reanimation 1250 year BC during the battle of Quadesh, but 3000 BC the "Kahein papyrus" mentioned already blood in urine and described a penis bamboo protection for bathing and swimming in the Nile (Fig. 8). It was suggested that "something"in the Nile waters was penetrating into the body

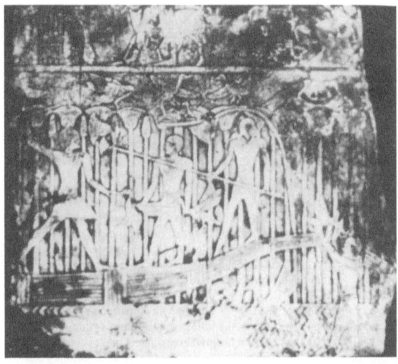

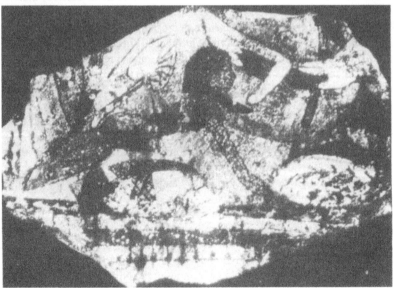

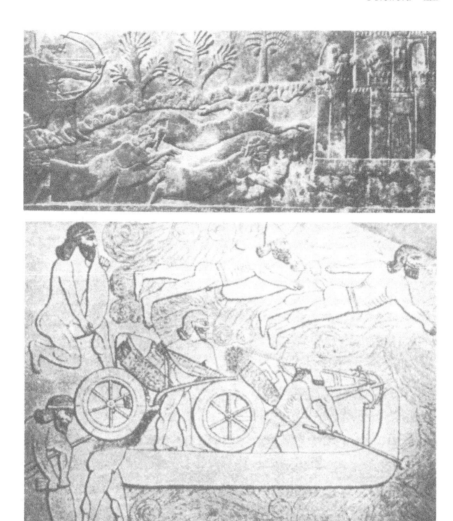

Fig. 2　Assyrian battle illustration (sculpturs and reliefs)
　　　　Swimming was essential for crossing waters with or without support
　　　　(900-600 B.C.) (4)

Fig. 1.　Egyptian swimming slave catching birds (1200-1100 B.C. - Egizio
　　　　Museum Torino) (5)

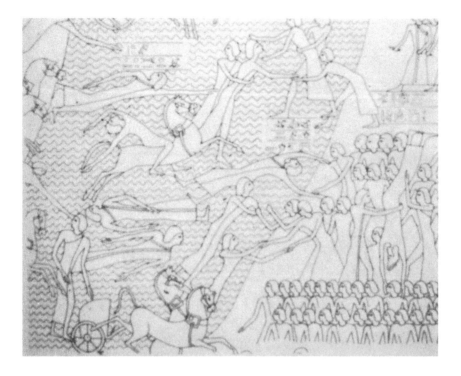

Fig. 3 Life saving, swimming and reanimation during the battle of
Quadesh(1250 B.C. - relief) (5)

▶

Fig. 4 Swimming in Greece : recreation or status ? (vases - 600-500 B.C.)
(1)

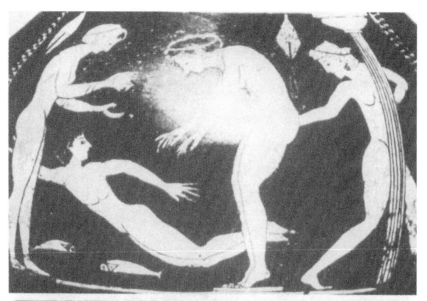

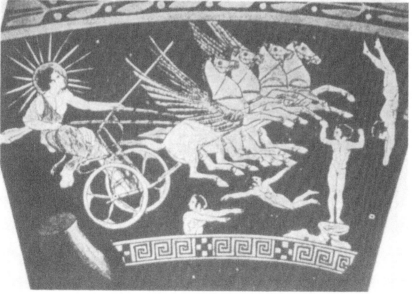

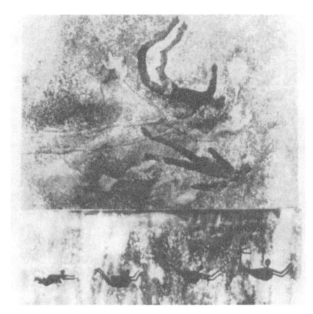

Fig. 5 In1933 the Frobenius expedition found different swimming figures
(paintings and carvings) in Nagoda, the bay of Kebir in Lybia (5000
B.C.) (2) A backstroke and a breaststroke are not imaginary.

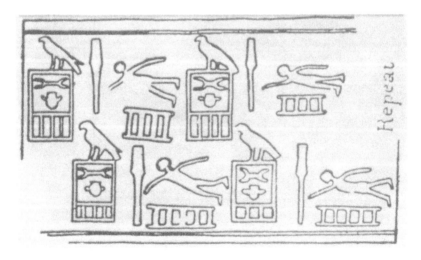

Fig. 6 Amongst the oldest hieroglyphes of the 2nd Egyptian dynasty a
side stroke or a crawl swimmer is represented several times (5000
B.C.)(6).

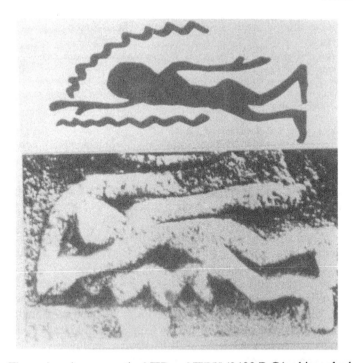

Fig. 7   The swimming man - the NEB or NEBU (2400 B.C.) a hieroglyph... of
the 6th Egyptian Dynasty (2)(7).

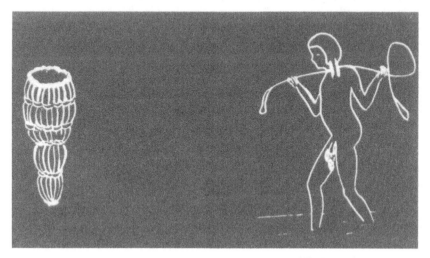

Fig. 8   Preventive Medicine... protecting the penis... avoiding
schistosomiasis (3000 B.C. and 1200 B.C.) (8).

(via the penis) creating gastrointestinal problems. The assumed problem was Schistosomiasis.

Schistosomisias is a worm (1 to 2 cm) that develops from (cercarian) parasites who live on snales in subtropical and tropical waters.

These parasites can penetrate the skin in a few minuts, go to the liver via the arterial system where they develop to worms who go and live and lay thousand of eggs in the colon, the ilium and the urinary bladder.

It is estimated that 200 million people have schistosomiasis (8).

Schistosoma eggs were found in mummies of 1200 BC.

We can assume that the associated gastro-intestinal problem explain why the several remainders of Egyptian swimming slaves were female.

Over the years and in comparison to other sports swimming has very little traumatic and/or clinical problems (9), but if problems there are, it are dominant shoulder problems.

According to Kennedy and Hawkins (1974) (10) shoulder pain appeared in Canadian swimmers for 3% only, while in American and European groups very different percentages were found (Richardson et al. 1980 (11) - 42%; Dominguez 1979 (12) - 50%; McMasters 1986 (13) - 68%). It is hard to believe that this variation is due to different swimming techniques. It is not known whether these groups had different training regimes. We do know that it occurs most in the frontcrawl, the backcrawl and the Dolphin. Its frequence is equal between males and females and it is mostly decribed as tendinitis, impingement syndrome and/or shoulder instability.

Shoulder instability can result from the joint and/or can be muscular in origin. Often the major complaint of the swimmer is : "My arm feels death... I have no strength in my arm..." this same complaint is often heard in patients with a thoracic outlet syndrome. In other words, a complaint that could find its origin in a compression of neuro-vascular structures also.

A cadaver study and in paralel an in vivo echographic study on 1321 military and sports men (N=1179) and women (N=142) confirmed the presence of the axillary Arch of Langer in 8.5% (male 8.39 and female 9.15%) (14).

This muscular arch of the axilla can be described as a little muscle coming from the M. latisssimus dorsi and joining the M. pectoralis major to insert on the lateral border of the sulcus intertubercularis of the humerus, thus passing medially to and in front of the Mm. biceps and coracobrachialis and the A. axillaris with the surrounding veins and nerves (Nn.medianus, ulnaris, radialis, cutaneus antebrachii medialis and cutaneus brachii medialis).

The axillary Arch of Langer (Fig. 9) will create a very specific compression of all nerves, veines and arterics entering the sulcus bicipitalis mediales resulting in a loss of strength during movements of the arm over 90° abduction ; 2/3 of the arm movement in all swimming strokes (except the breaststroke) is situated in that range of motion.

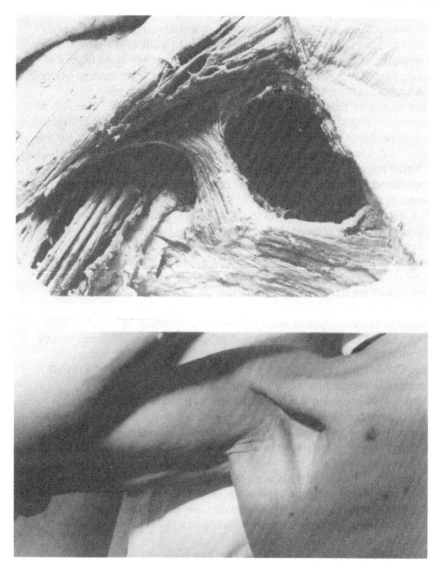

Fig. 9 The axillary Arch of Langer on cadaver and in vivo (14).

But there is more than swimming history, swimming culture and swimming medicine that leads to the science of swimming. Lewillie (1983)(15) stated : "Swimming as it is conceived today is a fairly new activity in the history of human kind". He herewith made allusion to swimming in the modern Olympic Games, but also to the pioneers of the science in swimming and interdisciplinary research such as DuBois-Reymond, 1905, 1927 (16) (17) ; Houssay, 1912(18) ; Liljestrand and Stenström, 1919 (19) ; Amar, 1920 (20) ; Hill, 1924 (21) ; Cureton, 1930 (22) ; Karpovich, 1933 (23)... and on. He was right : "...it is no older than one century".

During this century, a great deal of attention has been given to the pre-supposed relationship between body shape dimensions and hydrodynamic resistance (24)(20)(25)(26)(27)(28)(29)(30)(31)(23)(32)(19)(33)(34) (35)(36)(37)(38)(39)(40). However, only Clarys (25)(26) related drag for actively swimming subjects (active drag) to anthropometric variables. Contrary to expectations, Clarys (25)(26) found only few correlations between active drag and anthropometric variables, which forced him to conclude that the shape of the human body has hardly any influence on active drag and that other factors are therefore more important (41).

Given the fact that some argue that drag force is directly proportional to the product of velocity squared and a constant of proportionality, which among other things is dependent on the (projected) area of the body exposed to flow (42), one would expect at least some relationship between this variable and drag. The development of a new method of determining active drag (MAD system)(63) warranted a reevaluation of this relationship (41).

Hence what is needed in a interdisciplinary approach which combines hydrodynamic principles with anthropometric and morphologic knowledge in order to generate sufficient information to permit the study of drag created by the body form to propulsive drag in water which is created by human movement in water.

Assuming that active drag is one of the major components determining swimming performance, the hypohetical relation between body form and active drag should confirm (or reject) the idea that human body configuration is an accepted criterion for top swimmer selection or as influencing factors for performance ?

The question remains today : If the MAD hydrodynamic data of the eighties are correct ?! If the recalculations and renewed extrapolation of the Marine station data of the seventies indicate an over estimation !?... How will we explain that passive drag (Dp) and active drag (Ds) become not significantly different... with Dp and Ds having a very different turbulence.

Another question remains today : How do we relate a two dimentional antropometric depth, length, width, skinfolds value and their calculated ratio's with three dimentional but continuous changing and de facto unquantifyable body shapes during intensive swimming movement ?!

What are we doing ; do we need this ; do we not risk a proliferation of unproven or half proven facts...?

An example of similar and related nature : - In the literature, over 1000 articles can be found dealing directly or indirectly with skinfold measurements both in applied - including swimming - and fundamental research. Altogether more than 100 equations to predict "body fat" from skinfolds have been produced. The interest in skinfolds, given the easy accessibility of the subcutaneous layer and given its non invasive approach, has led to a proliferation of the commercialization and use of the skinfold caliper (43).

The available data have clearly demonstrated that skinfold compressibility is by no means constant. Adipose tissue patterning by assessment of skinfold thickness using calipers and incision confirms significant sex differences but emphasizes the neglected importance of skin thickness. It appears that the best adipose tissue predictors are different from those used in general. Also the problem of estimating body fat content by skinfold is compounded by the fact that two identical thicknesses of adipose tissue may contain significantly different concentrations of fat. Skinfolds are significantly related to external (subcutaneous) adipose tissue. However, the relation to internal tissue is less evident and the relation with intramuscular adiposity is unknown (44).

The relation of subcutaneous adipose tissue with the internal (intrathoracical - intraabdominal - intracranial) tissue is almost perfect in women and non significant in male (Fig. 10). In view of all this one of the miracles of contemporary science is how the linear distance between pressure plates of

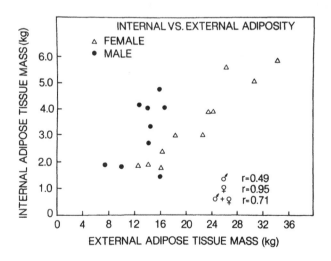

Fig. 10 The relation between external (= subcutaneous) and internal
human adipose tissue .

skinfold calipers is transformed into fat. In fact, when using skinfold calipers, what we are really measuring is the thickness of a double fold of skin and compressed external adipose tissue. To infer from this the mass of 'chemical' fat in the body requires a whole series of assumptions which cannot be supported by anatomical evidence.

Let us go back to the historical perspective and back to some of the physiology pioneers of the beginning of the century. In 1905 Du Bois-Reymond (16) and in 1919 Liljestrand and Stenström (19) studied cardiovascular and metabolic aspects of swimming. 1923, Alexander Hill (21) (the same Hill who received the nobelprize Medicine and Physiology in 1922) states that maximal performance in swimming is related to VO_2 max (21) and describes the role of lactic acid in the muscle after exercise. Up to the sixties it was difficult to determine lactic acid in blood, untill an easy enzymatic micromethod was found to assess the concentration of lactic acid which induced a spectacular proliferation of studies using arterial lactic acid to define the performance capacity. Most of these studies did not consider the basic principles of lactic acid metabolims and led therefore to a lot of controversies and contradictions. .. But advantaged too.

spiro-ergometry	lactic acid
- **complex and cumbersome equipment and measurement**	- **free sport practice (eg. no mask)** - **easy handling**

- **low resolution of precision**
- $\pm$ 0.81/min = $\pm$ 1.4ml/kg/min
  equivalence = $\pm$ 1.5s/100m
	- **high resolution of precision**
	- equivalence = $\pm$ .2mmol/1
	  = $\pm$ 0.25s/100m

- **maximal effort is necessary motivation is determining**	- **maximal effort is not necessary independent of motivation**

Lactic acid concentration in arterial blood is used to determine the physical capacity ; to define and adapt training intensities.

However it is imperative to avoid direct interpretation of lactic acid and one must look at the dynamics behind the lactic acid concentration, because we do not want a Rolls Royce to be equal to a Lada (...both have wheels, but...)

One lactic acid concentration at a given speed can be the result of many combinations of aerobic and anaerobic metabolic capacities.

Relations between speed and lactic acid depends on the form of exercise (e.g. modification of the exercise form induces another localisation of the "individual" aerobic threshold).

It is of crucial importance to know the exact aerobic and anaerobic metabolic capacity according to measure the lactic acid in order to ensure the validity of the assessment of the physical performance capacity of the swimmer and to determine his or her training intensity, quantity and form of exercise (45)(46).

Swimming Medicine, Swimming Hydrodynamics, Swimming Biomechanics, Swimming Physiology, Swimming Biochemistry... the step to Swimming Electromyography becomes easy. Strangely enough the pioneers of muscle electricity are amongst the oldest known scientists ever... the pioneers of swimming EMG are amongs the youngest

The pioneers of clinical and kinesiological electromyography are known to be Galvani 1792 (47), von Humboldt 1797 (42) and Duchenne (de Boulogne) 1855, 1862, 1867, 1872 (49)(50). A bibliometric survey of historical - if possible - original manuscripts have given a lot of informations on the works of different scientists related to Electrology or localizd electrization which became electromyography last century.

Among most scientists Galvani is considered the oldest source in electromyography (muscular irritation) but many original sources and correspondence indicate that many of his peers wereworking on the same topic before the major Galvani publication 1792 (47). In Belgium and Holland many anatomists and movement scientists know Swammerdam and Boerhaave (e.g. Kardel)(51) but very few know that Swammerdam discovered muscular electricity some 130 years before Galvani, who received the credit for it) (52).

Therefore it is very important at this point to acknowledge the work of Ikai and its coworkers 1964 (53) and of Lewillie 1967 (54) because they gave an unprecedented stimulus aswell. They measured EMG in water.No other sport has taken advantage of EMG since (Table1)(55).

Table 1 : Quantification (number of studies) of sport specific EMG research interest

swimming :	33	soccer :	3	Badmington :	1
cycling :	22	rowing :	3	Basketball :	1
running :	17	Judo :	3	Bowling:	1
skiing :	13	windsurfing :	2	cricket :	1
tennis :	8	archery :	2	FIN swimming :	1
gymnastics :	7	voleyball :	2	Handball :	1
Triple-hight-long jump :	5	baseball :	2	rifle shooting :	1
golf :	5	waterpolo :	2	sailing :	1
weight lifting :	5	Javelin :	2	skiff :	1
speed skating :	4	Kayak :	2	softball :	1
				synchro swimming :	1
				shot put :	1
				wrestling :	1

It remains very unfortunate however that some EMG studies cannot be used for comparison because of no or because of wrong normalisation techniques. The MVC is not the best choice as a reference (55).

Nevertheless EMG has become an important tool for obtaining muscle activity information, neccessary for the improvement of classical and alternative training methods (56)(55).

Let us summarize some of the most important findings.

- the trunk muscles during frontcrawl swimming have a significantly higher muscular intensity (IEMG) than any other muscle of the upper and lower limb. These trunk muscles make the difference between the elite and the good swimmers considering equal trainingsintensities.

Clearly and too often the importance of these back and abdominal muscles is underestimated. Additional and localized strength training is advisable.

- Dryland training devices - with or without accomodating resistance - are promoted (still) for their "movement specific workouts and strength increasing qualities". RMEMG and IEMG comparison with the "water" conditions have, however indicated that :

(a) there were overall time differences between dry land and "wet" arm cycle executions ;

(b) the muscle potential amplitudes were different in all five devices studied (expander, roller board, call craft, isokinetic swimbench and latissimus pull)

(c) most muscles showed fewer EMG peaks on dry land ;

(d) there were marked discrepanches for all comparisons (devices - muscles - functional groups - cycle phase separately) ;

(e) the dry land co-ordination creates a different pattern of movement.

It is generally observed that, whenever a swimmer acts against a mechanical resistance (especially in a different environment) important pattern deviation are noted. Specific training cannot be accomplished with dry land devices due to mechanical and environmental differences ((56)(57) In this case imitation does not mean specific.

Strength training effects are negligable or non existant because the intensities (IEMG) in dry land are inferior to those in water. Another study however, demonstrated similar relationship between stroke rate and VO2 max. in sprint swimming and during simulated all out swims on a isokinetc (or biokinetic) swimbench (58).

- Most commercial handpaddles produce specific activity, similar of "normal" swimming, but with higher intensities (IEMG). They are strengthening but place extra load on the shoulder also (59)(57)(60)(55).

Handpalm shaped paddles disturb the muscle pattern and have to be avoided.

- Tethered swimming is a recommended training method because of its highly specific muscular pattern at all velocities up to exhaustion (61). Semi tethered (with an allowed displacement of 8 m) is advisable for longer distance swimmers because at sprint speed the patterns are disturbed.

On the bases of IEMG values a strength training effect is suggested but not obvious.

- As to swimming (training) on the M.A.D. system (63) and in swimming Flume's - training De Luxe" - we know that different arm trajectories are inherent to both systems. In the MAD system because of pushing of on pads and in a Flume because of the laminar counter flow of the water. In both cases however the EMG patterns arrive at an acceptable level of specificity. The strength training efect again, maybe suggested but needs more study. Both the MAD system and the Flume however, are very valuable research instruments (62)((63)(64).

Strength training has become an important part of swimming training... but it is not sure that all trainers know what strength training is... or what can be done with it !?!?!!!!...
Strengh training... is more than increasing overall and local strength
* it is... agonist - antagonist ; concentric - eccentric ; constant - variable ; left - right... training
* it is monitoring and increasing muscular equilibrium.

In the past decade the development of dynamic muscle testing devices has increased our knowledge of the human neuromuscular system and its relation to performance, dramatically. The introduction of the isokinetic dynamometers based on the accomodating resistance principle allowing training and measurement of forces at a controlable constant speed throughout the range of motion. It gave a new impuls to the importance of strength training (65).
    The dynamic (isostonic) methods for strength training can fall into three categories : 1) constant, 2) variable, and 3) accomodating resistance (66). Numerous strength training machines have been developped as alternative to the traditional barbels and dumbbells, providing a more compact, convenient, and safer form of exernal loading. Their increasing application in all sports and swimming in particular has raised the inevitable question whether they are superior with respect to strength gain, and if they are, in what respect for each of the categories (67).
    In the constant resistance concept the load is always the same, i.e. a constant resistance through the total range of motion. Therefore, loading occurs at the weakest point in the system while the rest of the system is working at a lower capacity. To overcome this shortcoming, the variable resistance devices use pulley and cam systems and attempt to vary the resistance as the muscle lengthens or shortens. The reviewed litterature on strength training (65) indicates that both resistance exercise have seldom been compared, but when they have been studied neither method has shown overall superiority. Nevertheless, variable resistance devices may produce position-dependent increases which point to a specific training effect at the joint angle at which peak loading is induced by the device.

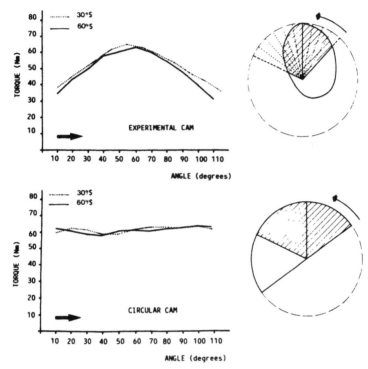

Fig. 11 The experimental cam for the variable resistance training and the circular cam design for the constant resistance training and their corresponding torque-angle curve patterns.

Pipes 1978 (66), De Witte et al.1988 (67) compared the effects of constant resistance training using a circular cam system versus variable resistance training, using an experimental cam design (Fig. 11), on the force angle relationship.

Without going into the detail of the concentric and eccentric work it is clear that both, constant and variable resistance training, increase strength significantly. The variable resistance mode, however, being the most profitable for both male and female, up to a very significant gain in female (Fig. 12) within a short (6 to 7 weeks) period of time.

The historical perspective of Swimming Science is like a very big house with many doors. We have used a few only, the house is big, very big, and very rich. Seven Int. Symposia on Biomechanics & Medicine in Swimming (WCSB)* plus ten World Congresses of Medical and Scientific aspects of aquatic sports (FINA)*

WCSB = World Commission of Sport Biomechanics ; FINA = Fédération International de Natation Amateur

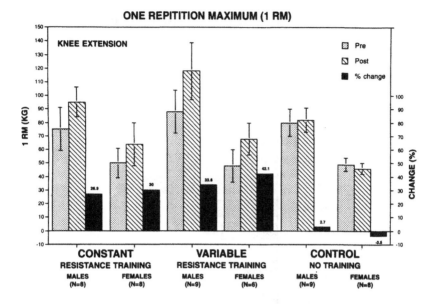

Fig. 12 Comparison of force scores, before and after variable & constant resistance extension at 60°/S and 30°/S for males and females.

has given us a wealth of research unique and unprecendented in the world of sports.

World FINA Medical Congresses

I	II	III	IV	V	VI
London	Dublin	Barcelona	Stockholm	Amsterdam	Dunedin
1969	1971	1974	1977	1982 with WCSB	1985

VII	VIII	IX	X	XI
Orlando	London	Rio Di Janeiro	Kyotō	Athene
1987	1989	1991	1993	1995

Biomechanics (& Medicine) in Swimming

1970	1974	1978	1982	1986	1990	1994
Brussels	Brussels	Edmonton	Amsterdam	Bielefelt	Liverpool	Atlanta

Research in Swimming

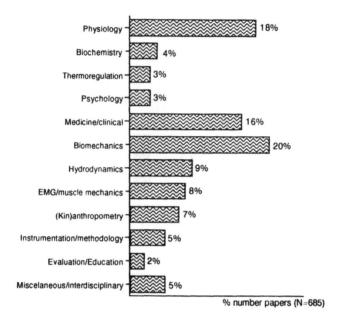

% number papers (N=685)

Fig. 13 Research topics in swimming expressed as percentage of peer
reviewed papers.

In addition and on the bases of peer reviewed papers swimming physiology
and biomechanics seem to have attracted the researcher most (Fig. 13) and
within these and other fields the front crawl received almost all attention. The
NEBU (Fig. 7) 2400 B.C. has shown the way.

References

1. Mehl, E. (1927) Antike Schwimmkunst, München, Heimeran Verlag.

2. Diem, C. (1960.) Welt Geschichte des Sports I en II, Stuttgart, J.G. Cotta'sche
   Buchhandlung,

3. Touny, A.D., Wenig, S. (1969) Der Sport im alten Agypten, Leipzig,
   Edition Leipzig.

4. Strommenger, E., Hirmer, M. (1964) Cinq millénaires d'art Mésopotamien, Paris, Flammarion.

5. Wenig, S. (1970) Die Frau im alten Agypten, Wien, München, Verlag Anton Schroll & Co.

6. De Villepion, G. (1929) Nageons, Paris, B. Grasset Editions.

7. Oppenheim, F. (1970) The History of Schwimming. North Hollywood, California 91607, Swimming World.

8. Girgis, R. (1934) Schistosomiasis, London, John Bale Sons and Danielsson, Ltd. publishers.

9. Merino, J.A., Llobet, M. (1978) Insertion tendonitis among swimmers in Swimming Medicine IV (eds. B. Eriksson, B. Furberg) Baltimore University Park Press, Vol. 6 pp. 101-104.

10. Kennedy, J.C., Hawkins, R.J. (1974) Swimmer's shoulder. Physician Sports Medicine 2, April, pp. 34-38.

11. Richardson, A.B., Jobe, F.W., Collins, H.R. (1980) The shoulder in competitive swimming. American Journal of Sports Medicine, Vol. 8 N°3, pp. 159-163.

12. Dominguez, R.H. (1979) Shoulderpain in age group swimmers. International Series on Sport Sciences; Vol. 6, pp. 105-109.

13. McMaster, W.C. (1987) Diagnosing swimmer's shoulder. Swimming Technique, february-april pp. 17-24.

14. Lafosse, F., Barbaix, E., Van Roy, P., Clarys, J.P., Van Rompuy, H. (1994) L'arc axillaire de Langer et son role possible dans le syndrome du défilé. Kine 2000, Vol. 5 N°4 pp. 29-33.

15. Lewillie, L. (1983) Research in swimming : Historical and scientific aspects. Biomechanics and Medicine in Swimming (eds. A.P. Hollander, P.A. Huijing, G. de Groot)Human Kinetics Publishers, Inc., Champaign, Illinois, pp. 7-16.

16. Du Bois-Reymond, R. (1905) Zur Physiologie des Schwimmens. Arch. Anat. Physiol. abt. Physiol.), Vol. 29 pp. 252-278.

17. Du Bois-Reymond, R. (1927) Der Wasserwinderstand des menschlichen Körpers. Pflügers Archiv. Physiol. Vol. 216 pp. 770-773.

18. Houssay, R. (1912) Forme, puissance et stabilité des poissons, Paris, Editions Herman et fils.

19. Liljestrand, G., Stenström, N. (1919) Studien über die Physiologie des Schwimmens (Studies on the physiology if swimming). Scandinavian Archives of Physiology, Vol. 39 pp. 1-63.

20. Amar, J. (1920) The human motor. London, Routledge and sons Ltd p.243.

21. Hill, A., Lupton, H. (1923) Muscular exercise, lactic acid and the supply and utilization of oxygen. Q.J. Med. Vol.16 pp.135-170.

22. Cureton, T.K. (1930) Mechanics and kinesiology of swimming. Res. Quart., Vol. 1 pp. 87-121.

23. Karpovich, P.V. (1933) Water resistance in Swimming. Res. Quart., Vol. 4 pp. 21-28.

24. Alley, L.E. (1949) An Analysis of resistance and propulsion in swimming the crawl stroke. Doctoral thesis. State University of Iowa, Iowa City.

25. Clarys, J.P. (1976) Onderzoek naar de hydrodynamische en morfologische aspekten van het menselijk lichaam. (Investigation into hydrodynamic and morphological aspects of the human body). Doctoral dissertation, Vrije Universiteit, Brussels.

26. Clarys, J.P. (1979) Human morphology and hydrodynamics in Swimming III (eds. J. Terauds & E.W. Bedingfield) Baltimore: University Park Press, pp.3-41.

27. Clarys, JP., Jiskoot, J., Rijken, H., Brouwer, P.J. (1974) Total resistance in water and its relation to body form in Biomechanics IV (eds. R.C. Nelson & C.A. Morehouse) Int. Series on Sportsciences, Baltimore, University Park Press, pp.187-196.

28. Councilman, J.E. (1951) An analysis of the application of force in two types of crawl strokes. Doctoral dissertation, University of Iowa, Iowa City.

29. Gadd, G.E. (1963) The hydrodynamics of swimming. New Scientist, Vol. 19 pp. 483-485.

30. Jaeger, L.D. (1937) Resistance of water as limiting factor of speed in swimming. Master's thesis, University of Iowa, Iowa City.

31. Jurina, K. (1972) Comparative study of fish man. Theorie Praxe Telesne Vychovy, Vol. 20 pp. 161-166.

32. Klein, W.C. (1939) Test for the prediction of body resistance in water. Master's thesis, University of Iowa, Iowa City.

33. Lopin, V. (1947) A diagnostic test for speed swimming the crawlstroke. Master's thesis, University of Iowa, Iowa City.

34. Miyashita, M. Tsunoda, R. (1978) Water resistance in relation to body size in Swimming medicine IV (eds. B. Eriksson, B. Firberg), Baltimore University Park Press, pp.395-401.

35. Onoprienko, B.I. (1967) Influence of hydrodynamic data on the hydrodynamics of swimmers. Theory and Practice in Physical Education USSR, Vol.4 pp. 842-847.

36. Safarian, I.G. (1968) Hydrodynamics characteristics of the crawl. Theory and Practice in Physical Education USSR, Vol.11 pp.18-21.

37. Schramm, E. (1960-1961) Die Abhängigkeit der Leistungen im Kraulschwimmen vom Kraft-Widerstand Verhaltnis. (The dependence of performance in the crawl stroke on the strength/resistance ratio). Wissenschaft Zeitschrift der Deutsche Hochschule für Korperkultur Leipzig, Vol. 3 pp. 161-180.

38. Tews, R.W. (1941) The relationship of propulsive force and external resistance to speed in swimming. Maser's thesis, University of Iowa, Iowa City.

39. Van Tilborg, L. Daly, D., Persijn, U. (1983) The influence of some somatic factors on passive drag, gravity and buoyancy forces in competitive swimers in Biomechanics and medicine in swimming (eds. A.P. Hollander, P.A. Huijing, G. de Groot) Champaign, Il., Human Kinetics, pp. 204-217.

40. Zaciorski, V.M., Safarian, I.G. (1972) Untersuchungen von Factoren zur Bestimmung der maximalen Geschwindigkeit im Freistillschwimmen (Investigations on factors determining maximal speed in freestyle swimming). Theorie und Praxis in Korperkultur Vol. 8 pp. 695-709.

41. Huijing, P.A., Toussaint, H.M., Mackay, R., Vervoorn, K., Clarys, J.P., de Groot, G., Hollander A.P. (1988) Active Drag Related to Body Dimensions in Swimming Science V (eds. B.E. Ungerechts, K. Wilke, K. Reischle) Human Kinetics Books, Champaign, Illinois pp. 31-38.

42. Rouse, H. (1946) Elementary mechanics of fluids. New York : John Wiley & sons inc.

43. Martin, A.D., Ross, W.D., Drinkwater, D.T., Clarys, J.P. (1985) Prediction of body fat by skinfold caliper ; assumptions and cadaver evidence. International Journal of Obesity, Vol.9 Suppl.1 pp. 31-9.

44. Clarys, J.P., Martin, A.D., Drinkwater, D.T., Marfell-Jones, M.J. (1987) The skinfold : myth and reality. Journal of Sports Sciences Vol. 5 pp. 3-33.

45. Mader (1984) Eine Theorie zur Brechnung der Dynamik une des steady state von Phosphorylierungszusland und Stoffwechselaktivität der Muskelzelle als Folge des Energiebedarfs, Deutsche Sporthochschule Köln.

46. Olbrecht, J. (1989) Metabolische Beanspruchung beiWettkampfschwimmern unterschiedlicher Leistungsfähigkeit, Stephanie Nagelschmid. Verlag Stuttgart.

47. Galvani, L. (1792) De Virbus Electricitatis in Motu Musculari.

48. von Humboldt, F.A. (1797) Versuche über die gereizte Muskel- und Nerven Faser. H.A. Rottmann,Berlin.

49. Duchenne (de Boulogne) GB. (1855, 1862, 1867) Physiologie des mouvements, Librairie JB Baillières, Paris.

50. Duchenne (de Boulogne) GB. (1872) De l'électrolisation localisée. Librairie JB Baillières.

51. Kardel, T. (1990) Niels Stensen's geometrical theory of muscle contraction (1667) : a reappraisal. J. Biomech.,Vol. 23 pp. 953-965.

52. Boerhaave, H., Gaubius, HD., Severinus, I., vander Aa, B., vander Aa, P. (1737) Joannis Swammerdammii Biblia Naturae ? Sive histoia insectorum, Leydae, .

53. Ikai, M., Ischii, K., Miyashita, M., (1964) An electromyographical study of swimming. Res. J. Phys. Educ., Vol. 7, pp. 47-54.

54. Lewillie, L. (1967) Analyse télémetrique de l'eloctromyogramme du nageur (Telemetric EMG analysis of the swimmer). Travail de la Société de Médecine Belge d'Education Physique et Sports Vol. 20 pp.174-177.

55. Clarys, J.P., Cabri, J. (1993) Electromyography and the study of sports movements : A review. Journal of Sports Sciences, Vol. 1 pp. 379-448.

56. Clarys, J.P. (1985) Hydrodynamics and electromyography : ergonomics aspects in aquatics. Applied Ergonomics Vol.16, N°1 pp.11-24.

57. Clarys, J.P. (1988) The Brussels swimming EMG project. In : B. Ungerechts, K. Wilke, K. Reischle (Eds.) Swimming Science V., Champagn, Ill., Human Kinetics, pp. 152-172.

58. Swaine, I., Reilly, T. (1983) The freely-chosen swimming stroke rate in a maximal swim and on a biokinetic swim bench. Medicine and Science in Sports and Exercise, Vol. 15 n°5 pp. 370-376.

59. Stoner, L.J., Luedtke, D.L. (1979) Variations in Front Crawl and Back Crawl Arm Strokes of Varsity Swimmers Using Hand Paddles in Swimming III (eds. J. Terauds, W. Bedingfield, R. C. Nelson, C.A. Morehouse) Int. Series on Sport Sciences, University Park Press, Baltimore, Vol. 8 pp. 281-288.

60. Monteil, K.M., Rouard, A.H. (1992) Biomechanical aspects of paddle swimming at different speeds in Biomechanics and Medicine in Swimming VI (eds. D. McLaren, T. Reilly, A. Lees) London, E. and F.N. Spon pp. 63-68.

61. Hopper , R.T., Hadly, C., Piva, M., Bambauer, B. (1983) Measurement of power delivered to an external weight in Biomechanics and Medicine (eds. A.P. Hollander, P.A. Huijing, G. de Groot) Human Kinetics Publishers, Inc. Champaign, Illinois pp. 108-112.

62. Holmer, I. (1983) Energetics and mechanical work in swimming in Biomechanics and Medicine in Swimming (eds. A.P. Hollander,P.A. Huying, G. de Groot) , Champaign, Illinois, Human Kinetics Publicers, pp. 154-164.

63. Hollander, A.P., de Groot, G., van Ingen Schenau, G.J., Toussaint, H.M., de Best, H., Peeters, W., Meulemans, A., Schreurs, A.W. (1986) Measurement of active drag during crawl arm stroke swimming. Journal of Sport Science, Vol. 4 pp. 21-30.

64. Hay, J.G. (1988) The Status of Research on the Biomechanics of Swimming in Swimming Science V (eds. B.E. Ungerechts, K. Wilke, K. Reischle), Champaign, Illinois, Human Kinetics Books, pp. 3-14.

65. Atha, J. (1981) Strengthening muscle in Exercise and Sports Science Rev. (ed. R.L. Terjung), Lexington : Collamore Press, vol. 9 pp. 1-73.

66. Pipes, T.V. (1978) Variable resistance versus constant resistance training in adult males. Europ. J. Appl. Physiol. Vol. 39 pp. 27-35.

67. De Witte, B., Claessen, L., Clarys, J.P. (1988) An evaluation of variable resistance exercise device in Biomechanics XI (Int. Series Biomech.) (eds. P. Hollander, G. De Groot, P. Huying, G.J. van Ingen Schenau), Champaign : Human Kinetics, pp. 1010-1015.

The author thanks Dr. Jan Olbrecht for the physiology information.

PART ONE

OVERVIEW

1 THE CONTINUUM OF APPLIED SWIMMING SCIENCE

J.P. TROUP
Keynote Presentation
VIIth International Symposium on Biomechanics and Medicine in Swimming

Abstract

Science plays an important role in the understanding and development of performance. Results from scientific studies can provide guidelines for training design, help determine performance potential and evaluate the training needs of athletes. The usefulness of science to the sport practitioner, however, is dependent upon the practical aspects of the research results combined with the ability of the user to understand basic concepts and limitations of science. Furthermore, it must be understood by both scientist and coach that any research study is only part of a scientific continuum; the ability to synthesize information from a wide variety of sources and study designs will determine how effective the practitioner can be when using science. Research represents the basic component in the learning process that includes a sequence of steps: presentation, demonstration and finally, application. With this approach, it becomes possible to evaluate, verify, reject, model and confirm concepts in training that may influence performance. This paper discusses the scientific continuum of applied science from the basic to highly practical aspects while reviewing the value and limitations of studies. Finally, project approach examples as models in the scientific continuum is presented.
Key Words: Swimming, Physiology, Coaching, Training, Education

1. Introduction

Over the years, and as the level of national and international swimming has become more competitive, sport practitioners have turned to science to help determine which training methods may be more effective than others. This is possible since science has played a role in defining categories of work and provided information on adaptations to different types of training (1,2,3). While this approach can be promising, its use has been limited by sport practitioners as the scientific basis for this information has been poorly understood. Often times this approach has led to high levels of frustration by coaches due to the inability of a single study to provide *the* answer as quickly as possible. The end result is that the value of science to the coach has been questioned, the information provided misused and/or misinterpreted and the type of scientific study conducted criticized. Why? Simply because the scientific process is misunderstood, the continuum of scientific research is overlooked and the importance of basic applied education is ignored. As a result, the need for sports science is questioned by coaches, practitioners and sports administrators. And rightly so since without addressing these basic issues, or establishing the key objectives for a program and clearly educating users of the approach and limitations, applied sports science programs will be of little measureable value to anyone.

The purpose of this paper, therefore, is to discuss 1) the continuum of science and its limitations in the pursuit of useful information based on the scientific process, 2) the sequence and evolution of events needed to establish a useful program and 3) examples of what is required to produce effective educational results and 4) to discuss recommendations for components of successful programs.

2. The Scientific Continuum

Coaches are routinely faced with four basic questions (1,2,3,) during the course of training design, including:
What to do, why, how and when.
This simple sequence of questions is illustrated by the need for developing endurance (*what*) for an athlete having poor performances (*why*) using long endurance sets with short rest intervals (*how*) at mid-season (*when*). The effective answer can be derived from the experience of trial and error, from reading papers, getting advice from other coaches, conducting studies or any combination of these sources.

The scientific approach can be used to minimize trial and error and help make sure that the selected training mode has the best chance of success(1,3,5,6). The area of greatest usefulness for sport science is in helping to answer the *what* and *how* of training. In the above illustration the critical concerns become understanding the most effective methods of developing endurance. In this case, the how becomes a question of determining whether a training set of 10 x 400 with 20 second rest intervals is better than 2 x (10 x 200) with 10 seconds rest, for example. The real advantage of science will come from conducting studies specifically designed to address training modalities and combination effects.

Determining the most correct answer will be dependent upon the total weight of evidence available. This is an important basic concept in the scientific process since no single study will provide *the* answer. Rather, the results from different scientific studies along with the results from practical experiences will help determine the best answer (3,4,5). This is illustrated by the following sequence of events:

The Learning Continuum

Scientific Results	Application	Evaluation	Improved Training

Furthermore, the results of any scientific study is limited (or strengthened) by:

1. The quality of design (i.e., study length, protocols, experimental groups, etc.),
2. The group participating in the study (i.e.,elite vs. average athletes; old vs young, etc.),
3. The use of specific test markers to measure an effect (i.e., performance, strength, etc.),
4. Influences of events that affect training or the experimental result,
5. Needed use of controls in the conduct of the study.

The scientific process is influenced by each of the above five points and is primarily influenced by point one (4). Study design must begin with identifying the problem and establishing a concept, or hypothesis, to test. The specific study design must be strong enough to properly answer the problem at a level that will reflect the conditions of the applied setting (3,4,5). Herein lies the biggest difference between basic and applied research; basic research requires that no outside influences be allowed that will have an impact on the results specific to the well defined experimental treatment. On the other hand, applied research can allow reasonable influences to be exerted on a study design (i.e., training studies) but only if they truely mimic the conditions that the user (i.e., coaches) will ultimately face in daily use of the information. For this reason applied programs will benefit most by using a process that provides for naturally occuring events to take place.

The scientific process does not differ at any level of design as it still involves testing a concept, quality controls in data collection, establishing levels of statistical significance, proper interpretation of data and explanation of results. Highly applied studies include each step but typically involves "free-living" populations rather than highly controlled laboratory conditions. With these studies the challenge of the investigator is to ensure that all subjects completed the requirements of the study so that the data interpretation is truely reflective of the condition being tested. This requires closer scrutiny and use of established standards that subjects must meet; if they are not met they should not be included in analysis so that the integrity of the design can be met. In contrast, highly controlled laboratory studies have no influences, subject compliance is typically not an issue so all data sets are consistently evaluated as part of the design. Both approaches will take time to conduct and evaluate and both will provide very valuable information - as long as the limitations and expectations of results are understood.

Following this approach, it should be clear that a continuum exists in the conduct of any study designed to demonstrate some type of an effect. The continuum can be represented by five levels on the basis of the extent to which scientific methods of design and control are possible or needed.

The levels of the scientific continuum presented in Figure One is reflect degrees of control. The studies having the most control (lack of external, influencing factors) are those that fit into Level One and Two. While these studies can be considered the most scientifically sound and are found in the most respected peer reviewed professional (i.e, scientific) journals, it is difficult to derive direct practical information that can be applied by coaches. Furthermore, if results are available only from these sources, coaches will never learn science. For this reason, other types of studies (i.e., Level three and four) are designed to build on the basic information provided from Level One and Two.

Figure One: Levels of The Scientific Study Continuum

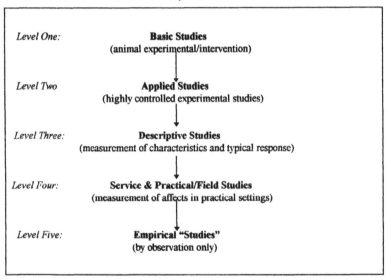

Studies within Level Three and Four represent important findings from a very practical and useful point of view while still maintaining scientific integrity and controls. Results from these study designs can be used to verify information from Level Two. An advantage of these levels is that they reflect the most typical training/living influences affecting the study population. The limitation of these studies, however, is the inability to tightly control confounding factors (coach/athlete compliance and cooperation) that may influence an effect. Any disadvantage that may be given up by not using the laboratory setting is made up by the usefulness of practical information derived from descriptive, practical studies. To this end when study findings of level three and four are combined with Level Two results, the coach is provided information as to whether a training design will actually work in a "free-living" condition. These studies can also be found in well-respected, peer reviewed publications and include symposium proceedings, annual research handbooks and smaller journals - all of which coaches and other sport practitioners have easier access.

Finally, empirical studies can serve as the final confirmation of results. Level Five studies however should never be used to demonstrate confirmation of a concept or answer a question but simply to confirm or reject the information collected as a final check. This is due to the fact that level five studies typically do not provide for a systematic comparison of a concept being tested at the same time under similar conditions. Furthermore, results can be influenced by personal bias since no statistical comparison is conducted.

In total, the levels of science in this continuum should be used as checks and balances. Such a system can be used to develop a theory, validate it, accept or reject it and, when appropriate, use it in training.

The successful use of science, then, does not come from one study, but several; it can not be done in one year but requires many to adequately answer and satisfy the question. If this is followed and the expectations of science made realistic, frustration levels can be kept to a minimum. Both coach and scientist must understand and accept that these levels of science properly exist.

2.1 Use of Appropriate Levels in the Continuum

Applied sport science programs should *primarily* address the concerns and needs of the sponsoring organization and its coaching community. Most sports organizations establish sports science programs to provide a service to coaches and athletes. It is critical that useful information is provided to the coach, enabling him/her to better understand the potential of the athlete being tested. This may be the single most important objective of a successful sports science program, provided that the test being administered is of practical and reproducable value.

A *secondary objective* must include the type of research that develops and validates a testing protocol and helps the sport practitioner understand its significance. Additionally, information must be collected through research to demonstrate what a specific test result means at a specific point in the training season.

The test protocol for the measurement of the anaerobic capacity developed at U.S. Swimming serves as an example. In this case, a research project was developed to first test the concept and, once proven, further research was conducted to determine how different training regimen would affect the value. Once satisfied with these results, descriptive data was collected to better understand how this value changes with the performance level of a swimmer.

This approach clearly demonstrates the use of a scientific approach and the importance of the continuum of science. Research is not conducted for research sake, but rather for a specific objective that will help enhance the knowledge base of the coach as a priority - not necessarily the investigator. Similarly, athletes are not tested just to be tested, but to add to the level of knowledge about a specific training concept. To this end, service is critical to sport science programming, not only to help evaluate athletes but to help educate athletes and coaches during cooperative efforts.

Finally, the *third* objective of a practical sport science program should be the conduct of research designed to model and evaluate <u>new</u> concepts in training. This objective in research, however, can only take place once the investigator understands how swimmers respond to training, why certain training regimen work and others do not and the current concepts in training are fully characterized and understood. Following this approach, other studies of an original nature should be conducted and driven by the interests and needs of the coach and athlete. Without this input, the scientist will be conducting research for research sake and address issues that are only of primary interest to the investigator. While academic research is important and can be helpful, any sponsored research project must address the practical issues that will have the greatest impact on swimming performance.

The best example of this challenge can be seen by looking at research results from average or below average swimmers that would suggest that athletes should train at low to moderate distance and fast paces. While this result may be true for some athletes at certain times of the season, empirical evidence demonstrates that it can not be true all of the time, particularly for elite highly trained athletes. In fact, most experienced coaches will argue that this latter approach to training is critical and that the other will not optimize performance. A lack of sensitivity to the scientific continuum without a balanced use of empirical evidence may result in false conclusions. This is an example of research for research sake at Level Two of the continuum but with a dangerous application.

In contrast, the approach used in practical sports science programs is one that tries to understand differences in training by first characterizing athletes in training and then montoring training with Level three and four studies. Researchers then discuss results with coaches for a perspective from Level five. From this, one can succesfully demonstrate how the economy profile of a swimmer changes, how it is influenced by training type and level, and why distance training actually enhances the ability to complete sprint training. This led to the realization that both distance training and event specific training were required at the elite level to enhance performance potential. This can only occur when a systematic, strategic approach is used.

An effective sport science program sponsored by sports organizations should focus on *Level Three and Four* studies as priorities. An appropriate balance of studies at *Level Two* should be conducted, but only as it will lead to the enhancement of service type programs. The benefit of this approach is that monies spent on programs will have the potential of directly benefiting the athlete as a priority, while providing the coach with hands-on educational opportunities. Those who lose sight of this need may conduct a few research projects each year that provide interesting reading, but little practical value. Once the academic community understands the need for this approach, research of greater benefit will be conducted and the scientific continuum within sports will become more effective.

3. The Evolutionary Process of Learning

Every applied sport science program encounters growing pains due to lack of understanding, frustration, jealousy, unclear goals and objectives. The normal development of these programs is an evolutionary process that takes years to successfully implement. By understanding this process and expectations it is possible to minimize some of the steps involved. The sponsoring organization demands demonstration of how sport science is affecting performance. Often the program must compete for funding or derive funding to support itself as well as other programs. Perhaps the largest challenge is one involving the lack of understanding of the continuum. Coaches, athletes and even those funding projects expect the results of testing or research even before that which can reasonably be expected. How can this process be minimized? The most important step, but yet often overlooked, is **education**.

Science requires a progressive approach to learning. It is not an easy discipline nor is it one that is appreciated overnight. Education is the cornerstone of every sport science program. Every cent spent on sport science is a waste of money for the individual who does not know how to apply the results of science. Without a strong education program, criticism of program expenditure for research and service is fair. The results of research are useless unless the end user understands the basic principles and limitations of science and how they can be used.

Table Two: Progression of exposure to science

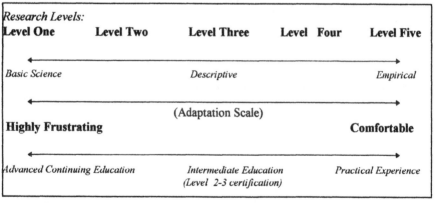

Even before the results of an active research program can begin, a basic education program must be in place. Such a program must include general and introductory concepts in swimming science including the disciplines of training, psychology, biomechanics and physiology. Only after some intermediate level of education is reached should continuing education take place that incorporates the presentation of current research findings.

Table two illustrates the need for a progression in education and use of science. As presented, first exposure to the scientific continuum results in an acceptable comfort level when limited to level five exposure. However, coaches will experience extreme degrees of frustration should higher levels be used before proper education takes place. Using science is very similar to understanding math. You cannot master multiplication without a sound understanding of basic addition. At each stage of learning the presentation of the basic concept must be made, followed by a demonstration of the concept which in turn is followed by a chance to apply the concept.

4. A Generation to Change and Adapt

Change will not happen over night or in a few years. This is most true when trying to implement programs that require education and practical experience. Effective change will take place, but it will require a willingness to go through those phases presented in Table Three and take up to 15 years to achieve. Currently, in the U.S. sport science is undergoing generational change and is somewhere between step 2 and 4 for the majority of users. The early years are often difficult but someone must pave the way so that it might eventually become easier for others.

Table Three: Steps involved in major professional change

Generational Steps to Change			
Steps in Change	*Timepoints in Change*	*Length of Period*	*Appropriate Research Level*
1. Want the Change	Due to lack of success	Up to a lifetime	Level 5
2. Frustrated by the Change	When realize change is difficult or don't understand	3 years	Level 3/4/5
3. Resist the Change	When habits must become different	3 - 5 years	Level 3/4/5
4. Think about the Change	When benefits result and start understanding	2 years	Level 2/3/4
5. Make the Change	When experience consistent success	2 - 6 years	Level 2/4
6. Sustain the Change	When experience steps 1 to 5	10 - 15 years	Level 1 to 5

It is often interesting to listen to those who criticize programs and suggest that sport science is responsible for the decline in performance levels of athletes. While sport science certainly deserves to be criticized for a lack of understanding or educational level, the implication that it is responsible for mediocre swimming is simply wrong. Misapplications can be blamed, but this is a result of not applying (or understanding) the correct pieces of information. In fact, the greatest benefit of science is that it should help organize a systematic approach to training. Clearly there must be some other reason that bad performances are experienced perhaps it is the result of an indivdual not familiar with sound principles of training. It's like blaming the library for doing poorly on an exam; the library, like sport science, is only a resource from which information can be gained. The bottom line is that the person on deck has to take the responsibility for not doing as good of a job as needed.

5. Model Approach Examples

Research plays an important role in identifying limiting factors of performance and developing methods to overcome them (1,3,4,5,6). An added benefit of research results is the information that can be added to educational materials. It is unfortunate, however, that few people realize the time and resources required to develop what may appear to be simple guidelines for training. As an example, in 1991 U.S. Swimming had developed a series of guidelines for interval training that included:

- Determination of ideal training distances for each category of work.
- Determination of the most appropriate rest interval for a type of training
           and selected interval distance
- Determination of ideal periods of training.

This information made significant contributions to our knowledge of interval training in that it took some basic empirical, unexpressed information from the coaching community and established very clear, concrete guidelines. In so doing the guesswork in training was minimized from previous generations of coaching resulting in more effective training regimen.

Although this looks simple, the final generation of this information require the following sequence of events:

1. Conduct studies which characterized the training status of highly trained swimmers.
2. Develop and test a protocol to measure the total energy demands of swimmers and devise an effective method of measuring energy contributions (aerobic vs. anaerobic)
3. Conduct a series of tests that describe the aerobic:anaerobic contributions of each competitive event.
4. Conduct studies to determine how these contributions are affected by training status and performance level of the athlete

5. Test different interval distances at various speeds using different work to rest periods and measure the aerobic:anaerobic contributions of each. Select the set design that most closely matches the energy profile described in number 3 above.

6. Conduct a training study comparing what and how adaptations are made with different interval training sets.

These series of studies took nearly three years to complete. The point of this description is to show that the scientific process does not happen overnight. It must be done in a systematic approach that includes problem identification using a subject population most closely matching those of interest to the organization. This is an approach that all sport practitioners must learn to appreciate if they are to interact with organizations that require practical information.

Similar approaches have been used in a variety of areas including age-group tracking and development, biomechanics, coaching skills, fuel use and psychology. Studies that can be used to improve performance must be conducted as a priority. Those studies that do not address this approach or are driven by individual investigator interest should not be supported.

6. Summary and Suggestions

Sports Science and Medicine can play an important role in the development and improvement of training and performance.

Prerequisites for this include:

1. recognition of the scientific process requirements
2. understanding the needs and interests of the coaching community (as priority),
3. accepting that a balance use of levels of scientific research is needed,
4. accepting that different levels of science are more appropriate in organized sports than in academic settings (i.e., Level 3/4/5 vs Level 1 and 2),
5. need to establish partnerships with various factions of sport practitioners so that the key users of the infomration generated will be part of the process,
6. implementing and meeting the critical need of basic education for sport practitioners,
7. ensuring a process for continuing education exists
8. continuous involvement of coaches in developing research directions,
9. accept the limitations and needs of the scientific process
10. be willing to accept and evaluate findings not allows matching preconceived thinking.

References

1. Bompa, T.A., Theory and Methodology of Training. Kendal/Hunt Publishing. Dubuque, IA. 1983.

2. Costill, D.L., E.W. Maglischo and A.B. Richardson. Swimming. Blackwell Scientific Publications. London, 1992

3. Maglischo, E.W. Swimming Even Faster. Mayfield Publishing Company Mountain View, CA, 1993.

4. Thomas, J.R. and J.K. Nelson. Research Methods in Physical Activity Human Kinetics Publishers, Champaign, IL 1990.

5. Troup, J.P. Research Annual 1992. United States Swimming Press. Colorado Springs, CO.

6. Troup, J.P. Research Annual 1991. United States Swimming Press. Colorado Springs, CO.

PART TWO
BIOMECHANICS

PROMETHEUS

2 CRITICAL ASPECTS OF BIOMECHANICS IN SWIMMING

M. MIYASHITA
Laboratory for Exercise Physiology and Biomechanics
Faculty of Education, University of Tokyo, Japan

Abstract
Biomechanical studies which were conducted by the author were reviewed in order to give effective advice to the swimming instructors and coaches pertaining to the hyperbolic relationship between swimming skill and energy yielding ability.
Keywords: efficiency increasing factors, energy increasing factors, swimming performance.

1 Introduction

Since 1967 when the First International Seminar on Biomechanics was held in Zurich, biomechanics in sports has been developed by numerous researchers of different backgrounds all over Europe, North America and many other countries.

Swimming has attracted the attention of many researchers with diverse scientific interests due to its unique nature. The author, along with many others, have conducted various research on swimming since 1960. The author believes that the research findings of sport biomechanics should be utilized to enhance athletic performance. In order to give effective advice to the swimming instructors, biomechanical findings must be rearranged by consulting the related physiological functions and growth and development.

The most popular way to give scientific advice to the coach is to point out the differences in performance and physical abilities between the highly-trained swimmers and untrained-swimmers.

1.1 Neuromuscular coordination in swimming strokes

To determine the pattern of timing and spacing of muscle activities in swimming, Ikai et al. [1]recorded EMGs of the arm, trunk and leg muscles during swimming of different strokes.

Based on the EMG recordings, they made the following conclusions; there was a common basic pattern of muscular activities in each type of swimming stroke; crawl, breast, back and butterfly strokes, respectively, the extensor muscles of the arm and the trunk were activated more vigorously to propel the body forward than the flexor muscles in the crawl, breast and butterfly strokes, with a slight exception in the back stroke, an elite swimmer was very skillful in activating major muscles during the stroking phase and relaxing these muscles during the recovery phase, compared with the middle-class swimmers.

1.2 Water resistance to body size

For example, in the case of same shaped ships, the bigger the ship, the greater the water resistance, and the bigger ship consumes a greater amount of gasoline than the smaller one, at the same cruising speed. In the case of human beings, however, it can be estimated from the data obtained by towing the swimmers, that water resistance encountered by the swimmer during swimming depends not only on body size, but on the body position to a wide range of body size. Therefore, it can be said that large, highly-trained swimmers are able to control their positions for reducing water resistance throughout their long-term practice in water.

1.3 Fluctuation of swimming speed during a single cycle stroke

The speed in the breast stroke during a single cycle stroke varies clearly from 0 to 1.2m/s in untrained swimmers and from 0.5 to 2.0m/s in highly-trained swimmers. The great decrease in speed is due to the recovery movements, by which both the knee and hip joints are simultaneously flexed [3].

On the other hand, in the crawl stroke, right and left arms and legs are moved alternately. Therefore, if the arms and legs of both sides are moved in good harmony, speed varies slightly during a single cycle stroke. Seven highly-trained swimmers swam 50m crawl stroke at their racing paces, and instantaneous swimming speed was recorded during three successive strokes. The mean speed of the three strokes of each swimmer ranged from 1.45 to 1.81m/s, and the amount of fluctuation of speed during a single stroke cycle ranged from 0.50 to 1.42 m/s among the tested swimmers [2].

Larger fluctuations of speed during a single cycle stroke must consume more energy. Then what percent of total work done in swimming 100m was devoted toward the speed fluctuation? In the case of a subject who had a Japanese record in the 100m free style, approximately 4% of the total work was calculated to be used for speed fluctuation. Moreover, if this extra energy could be used to propel the body forward, his record was estimated to be improved by 0.8s for the 100m.

1.4 Waves caused by swimmers

Previous experiments of water resistance indicate no significant difference in water resistance between static postures of small Japanese and large Caucasian top swimmers. Since physiological power is in proportion to muscle mass, small Japanese have to use physiological energy as effectively as possible. One example is how to minimize the fluctuation of swimming speed during a single cycle stroke as is described above. Another example is how swimmers acquire a swimming style which makes less waves. For that purpose, the amount of waves produced by self-moving swimmers was measured.

The measurements showed that the wave power (a square value of wave height per unit time) generally increased with swimming speed, and that the wave power at a given speed was lower in elite swimmers than in recreational swimmers. Therefore, wave power could be a useful parameter to identify the proficient level of swimmers [11,12].

1.5. Muscular force and swimming performance

Propelling force in swimming is produced by muscular activities. Arm-pull strength and speed of maximal swimming (crawl stroke) with arms alone were measured for 75 highly-trained male and female swimmers and 5 untrained male swimmers. There was a high positive correlation between arm-pull strength and swimming speed among the highly-trained swimmers. However, untrained male swimmers could not swim fast even though they possessed adequate arm-pull strength [4].

In addition, dynamic peak torque of the arm and leg were measured by a Cybex II on 35 swimmers of both sexes aged 11 to 21 years. These torques correlated significantly with the best records of a 100m free style, except between the peak torque of the knee extensor muscles and the best record of female swimmers [6].

Concerning this positive relationship between muscular force and swimming performance, the effects of strength training performed together with other swimming training were investigated. Eight male swimmers were tested before and after a 10 month training session. A significant correlation was obtained between gain in average peak torque for 100 repetitions of arm-pulling movement and gain in speed of 50m maximal swimming. Also all swimmers improved their racing times compared with those in the last session [7].

Elite and average competitive swimmers were tested in order to ascertain the relationship between starting performance and muscular force of the legs. There was a statistically significant positive relationship between diving distance from the starting block to the point where the swimmer's fingers entered the water and leg extension power in 69 swimmers using the crawl, butterfly and breast strokes. Also between the elapsed time from the starting signal to the moment when the swimmers head reached the 5m line and leg extension power in 57 swimmers using the crawl and butterfly strokes [9].

1.6 Aerobic power of competitive swimmers

The VO2max of elite Japanese swimmers in 1988 was compared with those of elite Japanese swimmers in 1968. World records improved 8 to 9% on average over the two decades from 1968 to 1988. The swimming speeds of Japanese elite swimmers were improved approximately 10% during the same period. However, there was no significant difference in mean VO2max between the two groups of elite swimmers in 1968 and 1988. Also, individual VO2max values of the swimmers who had qualified for the finals in both Olympic Games (in 1968 and 1988) were not clearly above the mean values of their respective groups [8]. The same results were observed on the Japanese female swimmers of 1992 Olympic Games [10]. These results suggest that VO2max was not a decisive factor for performance in swimming for elite swimmers who were homogeneous at an excellent level of VO2max (4.50l/min, 64ml/kg/min for males and 3.00l/min, 55ml/kg/min for females).

2 Summary

From the biomechanical and physiological point of view, maximal performance in swimming is mainly governed by two factors, viz., the maximal ability of the energy yielding process and the degree of efficiency (swimming skill). In other words, swimming performance is expressed as a hyperbolic relation between swimming skill and the energy yielding ability as is shown in Fig.1.

In the previous paragraphs, water resistance during being passively towed, speed fluctuation during a single cycle stroke, and waves produced by self-moving swimmers were reviewed as efficiency increasing factors, while muscular force (anaerobic energy production) and VO2max (aerobic energy production) were reviewed as energy increasing factors. For the purpose of instructing competitive swimmers successfully, other comparative research should be conducted from the viewpoint of growth and development.

The number of strokes and lap times for the first 50m of an official 100-m race were measured for elite older swimmers aged 16 to 24 years, and for younger swimmers aged 12 to 14 years. The same factors were measured for young beginners aged 7 to 12 years when they tried to swim 25m as fast as possible.

The average stroke time (Pt), the average distance covered in one stroke (Pd), and average swimming speed (V) were calculated.

In the case of the elite and young swimmers, there was a positive relationship between V and age. The increase in V depended mainly on the increase in Pd. Therefore, Pt remained almost constant over a large age range (from 12 to 24 years). On the other hand, in the case of young beginners both factors of Pt and Pd had an effect on the increase in V. These results suggest that the temporal pattern (rhythm) in swimming is obtained in the earlier stages of swimming practice.

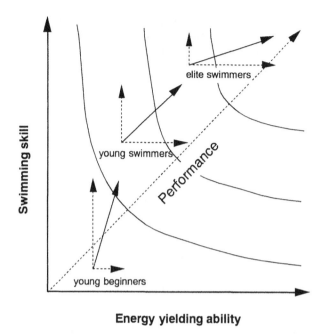

Figure 1. Hyperbolic relationship between swimming skill
and energy yielding ability

Young beginners (under 10 years of age) are able to swim at a certain speed as a result of their great improvement in swimming skill despite their relatively limited physical ability. This may be supported by the results that young beginners improve their swimming performance by rapid acquisition of the temporal pattern of arm action.

As for the young swimmers (teenagers), their swimming performance is greatly improved year-by-year with swimming practice, in addition to natural growth and development. On the contrary, the improvement of swimming performance of elite swimmers is dependent only on the development of both their aerobic and anaerobic energy yielding abilities through hard training, such as weight training, interval training, etc.

Thus, researchers of biomechanics who wish to communicate their research findings to sport coaches successfully, should take into account the physical ability to exert energy. For understanding this relationship more clearly, swimming performance should be expressed as a hyperbolic function of neuro-muscular efficiency and energy yielding ability, as is indicated in Fig.1.

Since both energy yielding ability and neuromuscular coordination develop with age, age-related approaches are indispensable in biomechanics in swimming. In other words, biomechanists in swimming should assess both the swimming performance from the kinematic and kinetic points of view and the maximal ability of energy output of the athlete in order to realize his/her swimming performance totally.

3 References

1.   Ikai, M. Ishii, K. Miyashita, M. (1964) An electromyographic study of swimming. *Japan Journal of Physical Education*, Vol. 7, pp. 47-54.

2.   Miyashita, M. (1971) An analysis of fluctuations of swimming speed. *In First International Symposium on Biomechanics in Swimming, Waterpolo and Diving* (ed. L. Lewillie & J.P. Clarys) , pp. 53-57, Universite Libre de Bruselles.

3.   Miyashita, M. (1974) Method of calculating mechanical power in swimming the breast stroke. *Research Quarterly*, Vol.45, pp.128-137.

4.   Miyashita, M. (1975) Arm action in the crawl stroke. *In Swimming II*. (ed. L. Lewillie & J.P. Clarys), Baltimore, University Park Press, pp. 167-173.

5.   Miyashita, M. Tsunoda, T. (1978) Water resistance in relation to body size. *In Swimming Medicine IV*, (ed. B. Erikson & B. Furberg), Baltimore, University Park Press, pp. 395-401.

6.   Miyashita, M. Kanehisa, H. (1979) Dynamic peak torque related to age, sex, and performance. *Research Quarterly*, Vol. 50, pp. 247-255.

7.   Miyashita, M. Kanehisa, H. (1983) Effect of isokinetic, isotonic and swim training on swimming performance. *In Biomechanics and Medicine in Swimming*, (ed. A.P. Hollander, P.A. Huijing & G. de Groot G), Champaign, Human Kinetics, pp. 329-334.

8.   Miyashita, M (1989) Cross-sectional comparison of maximal oxygen uptakes of Japanese elite swimmers with 20 years intervals. *Japanese Journal of Sports Sciences*, Vol.8, pp. 707-710.

9.   Miyashita, M. Takahashi, S. Troup, J. P. Wakayoshi, K. (1992) *Leg extension power of elite swimmers. In Biomechanics and Medicine in Swimming*, (ed. D.Maclaren, T. Reilly and A. Lees), E & FN Spon, London, pp.295-299.

10.   Miyashita, M. Mutoh, Y. (1994) A comparison of maximal aerobic power of Japanese elite female swimmers. *Coaching and Sport Science Journal*, Vol.1, pp.19-22.

11.   Ohmichi, H. Takamoto, M. Miyashita, M. (1983) Measurement of the waves caused by swimmers. *In Biomechanics and Medicine in Swimming*, (ed. A.P. Hollander, P. Huijing & G. deGroot), Champaign, Human Kinetics, pp. 103-107.

12.   Takamoto, M. Ohmichi, H. Miyashita, M. (1983) Wave height in relation to swimming velocity and proficiency in front crawl. *In Biomechanics IX-B*. (ed. D.A. Winter, R.W. Norman, R.P. Wells, K.G. Hayes & A.E. Patle), Champaign, Human Kinetics, pp. 486-491.

3 SOME ASPECTS OF BUTTERFLY TECHNIQUE OF NEW ZEALAND PAN PACIFIC SQUAD SWIMMERS

R.H. SANDERS
School of Physical Education
University of Otago, Dunedin, New Zealand

Abstract
The purpose of this study was to quantitatively analyze the techniques of New Zealand's most elite butterfly swimmers. Four male and three female New Zealand Pan Pacific Squad members who race in butterfly and/or individual medley were requested to swim butterfly at race pace. Two PAL video cameras simultaneously recorded the above and below water views perpendicular to the line of travel of each swimmer. Paths of the vertex of the head, shoulders, hips, knees, ankles, and feet were obtained by digitizing the video records. Center of mass, stroke length and stroke frequency, and trunk and thigh angles were computed. Center of mass velocity and acceleration were derived from the Center of mass record. Unlike the findings for a similar study of breaststroke technique, stroke lengths and stroke frequencies varied within a relatively small range. Differences among the subjects were most apparent in the center of mass velocity and acceleration profiles. In particular, swimmers varied in the relative magnitudes of propulsive accelerations associated with the phases of the pull and kick. There was a considerable vertical undulation of the CM for both males (approx 18 cm) and females (approx 14 cm). This finding, together with the shoulder and hip path data, is contrary the belief held by many coaches that center of mass undulations are minimized by out of phase undulations of the hips and shoulders.
Keywords: Butterfly, swimming, technique.

1 Introduction

Studies of Olympic Games performances have shown that elite butterfly swimmers vary considerably with respect to basic kinematic variables such as stroke length and stroke frequency [1]. For example, it has been found that more successful butterfly swimmers tend to have longer stroke lengths and slower stroke frequencies than less successful swimmers.

Quantitative analysis of the vertical motions of butterfly swimmers has indicated that the vertical undulations of the body during the butterfly stroke cycle are sequenced so that a body wave travels in the cephalo-caudal direction and contributes to a whip-like kick [2]. Consequently, the magnitude and timing of these undulations affects performance. That study indicated that, even at the most elite level, there is substantial variability in technique among swimmers.

Quantitative data on elite butterfly swimming remains sparse for some important kinematic variables. Thus, the purpose of this study was to quantitatively analyze the techniques of New Zealand's most elite butterfly swimmers.

2 Method

Four male (M1, M2, M3, M4) and three female (F1, F2, F3) New Zealand Pan Pacific Squad members who race in butterfly and/or individual medley participated in this study. Swimmers were marked with black tape at points in line with the shoulder, elbow, wrist, hip, knee, and ankle axes of rotation. Scale lines with markers at 50 cm intervals were stretched tightly above and below the swimmers' line of motion. These were placed seven lanes away from the cameras.

The swimmers were requested to swim at race pace through the recording area. One Panasonic M40 standard PAL video camera and one Panasonic M7 standard PAL video camera simultaneously recorded the above and below water views of the swimmers from the side at 50 fields per second. The cameras were panned to maximize image size.

The above and below water views were digitized on a PEAK Performance 2D digitizing system. Bilateral symmetry was assumed and only the camera side of the body was digitized to define an eight segment body model comprising head and neck, trunk, arms, forearms, hands, thighs, shanks, and feet. The raw digitized points from the above and below views were then scaled, aligned using the known positions of points digitized from the scale lines, and combined to produce coordinates for the whole body using a FORTRAN program. Center of mass (CM) was determined by applying the anthropometric data of Dempster [3]. Data corresponding to one stroke cycle, defined as the period from the instant of wrist entry to the next, were then analyzed. Cycles in which the camera axes were close to perpendicular to the swimming direction were selected for analysis.

The variables quantified in this study were stroke length, stroke frequency, the timing of the pull, recovery, and the downbeats of the two kicks, CM velocity and acceleration in the swimming direction (horizontal), and vertex, shoulder, hip, CM vertical range of motion.

3 Results

3.1 Stroke length and stroke frequency.

Table 1 shows stroke frequency, stroke length (horizontal distance travelled by the CM during the cycle) and the average CM horizontal velocity over the cycle. The male and female subjects are listed in order of average CM velocity (M1, M2, M3, M4, F1, F2, F3). It should be recognized that the swimmers were not racing and that the differences between adjacent rankings were smaller than the likely errors in the measurements. The 1988 Olympic gold medal winning performances of Anthony Nesty and Kirsten Otto in the first 50 m of the 100 m are provided for comparison.

Table 1.   Stroke frequency, stroke length, and average CM horizontal velocity

Swimmer Velocity	Stroke frequency (cycles/s)	Stroke length (m)	Av. CM (m/s)
M1	0.88	1.86	1.63
M2	0.71	2.26	1.62
M3	0.80	1.98	1.58
M4	0.87	1.77	1.54
F1	0.91	1.61	1.46
F2	0.77	1.74	1.34
F3	0.78	1.69	1.32
Nesty [1]	0.86	2.16	1.86
Otto [1]	0.97	1.75	1.70

Swimmer M2 had the smallest stroke frequency (0.71 cycles/s) and the longest stroke length (2.26 m) of all the squad members. The stroke lengths of M2 are comparable to those of Anthony Nesty (2.16 m). However, the stroke frequency was less than that of Anthony Nesty (.86 cycles/s). Swimmer M1 had CM velocity (1.63 m/s) similar to that of M2. However, M1 relied on a higher frequency (.88 cycles/s) than M2 and had a smaller stroke length (1.86 m). This difference in stroke length/stroke frequency was probably partly related to body length with the shorter swimmer (M1) having a shorter stroke length and higher frequency. The stroke frequency of M1 was similar to that of Anthony Nesty but stroke length was considerably less.

The fastest female (F1) had the highest stroke frequency (0.91 cycles/s) and the shortest stroke length (1.61 m) of all the squad swimmers. These frequencies approached those of Kirsten Otto (0.97 cycles/s). Her stroke length was less than Kirsten Otto's (1.75 m).

3.2 CM horizontal velocity

Maximum velocities of the group ranged from 1.84 m/s (F2) to 2.23 m/s (M1). Minimum velocities ranged from 0.52 m/s (F3) to 1.22 m/s (M1). Swimmer F3 had the largest range (1.40 m/s) of CM horizontal velocity reaching a minimum of 0.52 m/s. This would be expected to incur a large metabolic cost in accelerating back to top speed. Swimmer F2 also had a large fluctuation in velocity (1.28 m/s) with the minimum being (0.57 m/s). The other swimmers had ranges of approximately 1 m/s. It is noteworthy that M2 had the least fluctuation (0.92 m/s) despite having the smallest frequency. This indicated good streamlining during the non-propulsive phases.

The group was split with respect to the timing of maximum velocity. Four of the seven squad members M2, M4, F1, F3 attained the greatest velocity towards the end of the stroke cycle corresponding to the finish of the backsweep combined with the second kick. Swimmers F3 and M1 attained their greatest velocities during the first kick. Swimmer M3 attained a maximum velocity during the outsweep.

The time of attainment of the lowest velocities varied substantially among the swimmers from prior to hand entry to the commencement of the insweep. Figure 1 shows the CM velocity profiles of M2 and F2. Differences in the profiles indicate the typical variability among the subjects in terms of the range of velocity and the actions which generated the greatest change in velocity (propulsion).

3.3 CM Acceleration

The patterns of CM acceleration varied considerably reflecting differences in the phases of the stroke that were the most propulsive. Swimmers F2 and F3 had a strong first kick. Swimmer M1 had a strong first kick but also had a strong backsweep combined with the second kick. Swimmer M3 had a strong outsweep and backsweep/second kick. Swimmer M4 relied mostly on a strong backsweep combined with second kick. Swimmer F1 had major contributions to propulsion from the insweep and backsweep combined with the second kick. Her decelerations were small indicating efficient technique and streamlining. Swimmer M2 gained propulsion mainly from the first kick and early in the insweep. Like F1 his accelerations and decelerations were confined within a relatively small range indicating economical technique.

3.4 Vertex, shoulder, hip, and CM undulations

The range of vertical undulations for the vertex, shoulder, hip, and CM are shown in Table 2.

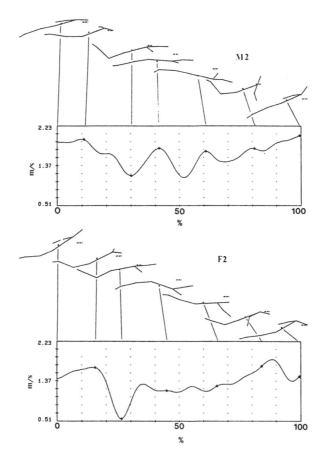

Fig. 1.   CM velocity profiles of M2 and F2 over one stroke cycle

Table 2.   Vertical undulations

Swimmer CM (cm)	Vertex (cm)	Shoulder (cm)	Hip (cm)	
M1	51	35	21	16
M2	58	43	13	19
M3	62	40	16	19
M4	63	40	16	18
F1	45	36	11	14
F2	70	38	18	13
F3	51	32	9	14

The undulations were substantial for all swimmers. The shoulder undulations were between 32 cm (F3) and 43 cm (M2). The hip undulations were considerably less than the shoulder undulations being between 9 cm (F3) and 21 cm (M1).

The male swimmers had CM undulations between 16 cm and 19 cm and the female swimmers had CM undulations of 13 cm to 14 cm. The relatively large CM undulations supported the suggestion that raising the CM and reusing the accrued energy using a body wave action contributes to propulsion [2]. It was also interesting that the swimmers with the smallest variation in CM velocity (M2 and M3) had the largest amplitude of CM undulation while the swimmers with the smallest CM undulation (F2 and F3) had the largest variation in CM velocity.

4 References

1. Nelson, R.C., Brown, P.L., Kennedy, P.W., Chengalur, S.N. (1988) *An Analysis of Olympic Swimmers in the 1988 Summer Games.* Biomechanics Laboratory Pennsylvania State University.

2. Sanders, R.H., Cappaert, J.M., Devlin, R.K., and Troup, J.P.(1992) Evidence of energy reuse through body wave motion in butterfly swimming. (eds. R. Rodano, G. Ferrigno, G. Santambrogio), *Proceedings of the 10th Symposium of the International Society of Biomechanics in Sports.* Edi.Ermes Milano, pp.67-70.

3. Dempster, W.T. (1955) *Space Requirements of the Seated Operator.* (WADC TR 55-159), Wright-Patterson Air Force Base, OH.

4 ROTATIONAL BALANCE ABOUT THE CENTER OF MASS IN THE BREASTSTROKE

J.M. CAPPAERT
U.S. Swimming, International Center for Aquatic Research
University of Colorado, Colorado Springs, USA

Abstract
The purpose of this study was to evaluate angular momentum about a breaststroker's center of mass. Breaststrokers (n=8) were filmed using a four camera system at the 1992 Olympic Games during the men's 200m preliminary and final races. Two cameras in underwater housings were placed on the floor of the pool underneath each laneline defining lane four. Two cameras were placed 5m above the water (attached to the 50m wall) on both sides of lane 4. These cameras were focused downward toward the center of lane four at the 45m mark of the pool. All four cameras had the same view of the swimmer during the competition. The videotapes were digitized to construct a three-dimensional (DLT method) 14 segment rigid model. The center of mass was calculated and displacement data were differentiated. Local angular momentum of the segments and their remote angular momentum about the body's center of mass was calculated (Dapena, 1978). Angular momentum data were not significantly correlated with swimming velocity, but elite level breaststrokers were more symmetrical than less elite athletes.
Keywords: Angular momentum, breaststroke, symmetry.

1 Introduction

The purpose of this study was to describe the center of mass and the segmental angular momentum in the breaststroke. It was hypothesized that swimmers with better balance of clockwise (CW) and counterclockwise (CCW) angular momentum about the three cardinal axes would be more efficient and would be the fastest swimmers.

2 Methods

2.1 Subjects
The subjects included eight male breaststrokers participating in six preliminary heats, the consolation final and the championship final of the 1992 Olympic Games. Subjects had a range of swim velocities from 1.2 to 1.6 m/s (mean = 1.45 ± 0.11m/s). Swimmers in the first four preliminary heats were not elite level breaststrokers as compared to the remaining four swimmers which included the world record holder for this event. Each athlete's height and weight was gathered from the Olympic athlete database.

2.2 Video Recordings
During each preliminary heat and the two finals, the swimmer in lane 4 was recorded using a four camera system. Two cameras in underwater housings were placed on the floor of the pool underneath the lanelines defining lane 4. The optical axes of the cameras were focused upward and toward the center of the lane. Swimmers were videotaped as they swam toward the 50m wall at the 40-45m mark of the pool.

Two cameras were placed 5m above the water surface. The optical axes of these two cameras were focused downward toward the center of lane 4. These two cameras also videotaped the swimmers at the 40-45m mark. Therefore, all four cameras recorded the same position in the pool and the same stroke cycle of the swimmers. The Direct Linear Transformation method (Abdel-Aziz and Karara, 1971) was used for three-dimensional analysis. This analysis was performed separately in the over and underwater camera sets.

2.3 Videotape Digitizing
Twenty-four body landmarks were digitized using the two underwater videotapes for one complete stroke cycle to create a fourteen segment rigid model. During out of water motions, the two over water videotapes were used for digitizing. Three-dimensional under and over water coordinates were calculated separately. All coordinates were then expressed in terms of a reference frame in which the X-axis defined the forward swim direction, the Y-axis defined the sideways direction and the Z-axis was vertical.

2.4 Data Calculations
The center of mass was calculated (Dempster, 1955) and displacement data were smoothed using a low-pass Butterworth filter (6 Hz) and differentiated. Total angular momentum about the body's center of mass was calculated using a method developed by Dapena (1978). This method computes a local and remote angular momentum term for each body segment. Segmental contributions to the total body angular momentum were evaluated.

3 Results

Angular momentum about the center of mass during a complete stroke cycle is represented in Figure 1. Average maximum clockwise and counterclockwise values (Table 1) were similar within the group of breaststrokers. Maximum and minimum segmental contributions to the center of mass angular momentum are presented in (Table 2).

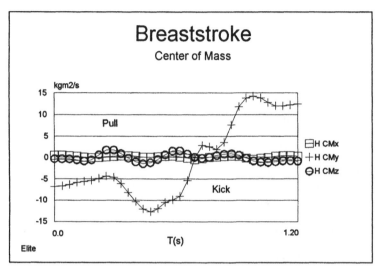

Figure 1: Angular Momentum Values of the Center of Mass about the X-axis (front view), Y-axis (side view), and Z-axis (overhead view).

Table 1: Angular Momentum Data of the Center of Mass about the X-axis, Y-axis, and Z-axis.

Variable	Mean	(Std)
Maximum CW about Y-axis (kgm^2/s)	-13.3	(3.3)
% of stroke cycle that max CW occurs about Y-axis (%)	38.3	(2.6)
Maximum CCW about Y-axis (kgm^2/s)	12.8	(3.0)

% of stroke cycle that max CCW occurs		
about Y-axis (%)	80.6	(10.4)
Average about X-axis (kgm^2/s)	0.3	(0.3)
Average about Z-axis (kgm^2/s)	-0.6	(0.4)

Table 2:   Maximum Counterclockwise (CCW, positive values) and Clockwise (CW, negative values) Angular Momentum Data of the Body Segments about the X-axis, Y-axis, and Z-axis.

Variable	Mean	(std)
Right Arm		
About X-axis (kgm^2/s)	1.3	(0.3)
About Y-axis (kgm^2/s)	1.2	(0.4)
About Z-axis (kgm^2/s)	-3.3	(0.8)
Left Arm		
About X-axis (kgm^2/s)	-1.3	(0.2)
About Y-axis (kgm^2/s)	1.5	(0.3)
About Z-axis (kgm^2/s)	3.3	(0.7)
Right Leg		
CW About Y-axis (kgm^2/s)	- 4.0	(1.1)
CCW About Y-axis (kgm^2/s)	4.7	(1.1)
About Z-axis (kgm^2/s)	-7.2	(1.5)
Left Leg		
CW About Y-axis (kgm^2/s)	-4.0	(1.0)
CCW About Y-axis (kgm^2/s)	4.2	(1.2)
About Z-axis (kgm^2/s)	6.8	(1.1)
Head CW about Y-axis (kgm^2/s)	-3.2	(0.8)
Head CCW about Y-axis (kgm^2/s)	2.7	(0.7)
Trunk CW about Y-axis (kgm^2/s)	-2.5	(0.6)
Trunk CCW about Y-axis (kgm^2/s)	2.0	(0.4)

4 Discussion

The center of mass data about the Y-axis (the angular momentum values about the X- and Z-axes were very close to zero, Table 1) showed a larger CW (motion upward to breathe) than CCW. The head and trunk about the Y-axis mimicked the center of mass data. Together these data may suggest that breaststrokers emphasize the upward motion to breathe rather than the downward diving motion to begin the pull.

The group of eight breaststrokers were very symmetrical in their segmental contributions to the total angular momentum about the center of mass (Table 2). In general, the right and left arms had almost equal and opposite angular momentum values about the three axes. The legs showed slight asymmetries about the Y- and Z-axes suggesting that the kick may be less efficient than the arm pull. This inefficiency in the legs may be due to the lack of visual cues as to the positioning of the legs during the kick.

Although none of the calculated variables were significantly correlated to swimming performance, elite level breaststrokers were more symmetrical than non-elite breaststrokers especially in the legs during the kick. The slowest swimmer of the group had large maximum angular momentum differences about the Z-axis during the kick (-9.7 vs. 5.3 kgm^2/s, right and left legs respectively), whereas the fastest four swimmers had similar and opposite amounts.

5 References

1.   Abdel-Aziz, Y.I. and Karara, H.M. (1971) Direct linear transformation: From comparator coordinates into object coordinates in close-range photogrammetry. *Proceedings ASPUI Symposium on Close-Range Photogrammetry*. American Society of Photogrammetry, Church Falls, VA, pp. 1-19.

2.   Dapena, J. (1978). A method to determine the angular momentum of a human body about three orthogonal axes passing through its center of gravity. *Journal of Biomechanics*, 11:251-256.

3.   Dempster, W.T. (1955). Space requirements of the seated operator, *WADC Technical report*, Wright-Patterson Air Force Base, Ohio.

5 HAND FORCES AND PHASES IN FREESTYLE STROKE

A.H. ROUARD*, R.E. SCHLEIHAUF**
and J.P. TROUP***
*Centre de Recherche et d'Innovation sur le Sport, Lyon, France
**Hunter College, New York, USA.
***U.S. Swimming, University of Colorado, Colorado Springs USA.

Abstract
The aim of the study was to examine times and forces distributions through the different phases of the freestyle stroke cycle and the influence of the level of performance on these parameters. Nine males ranging from local to international level of performance swam 4x25m in freestyle at a common speed (1.6 m/s). From the digitizing side and front video views, kinematic parameters were used to calculate hand forces according to Schleihauf's method. The integrals of the lift-drag-resultant forces and projection of the resultant on the forward axis were expressed for the aquatic part of the stroke and 4 phases (P1 :arm-trunk angle 0°to30°, P2:30°to90°, P3:90°to135°, P4:135°to180°). Results indicated longer first phase and greater forces production for the final phase as mentioned in previous studies. Large individual variations were noted for all the studied parameters. Poor correlations were obtained between the forces-times distributions through the phases and the level of performance. For the studied speed, best swimmers differed only for the final phase, presenting shorter duration and higher forces.
Keywords: freestyle, hand, forces, performance, speed.

1 Introduction

Since the beginning of the 20th century, many authors have tried to measure the forces using different methods. The tethered swimming has been the first used by Houssay [1], Cureton [2], Karpovich and Pestrecov [3]. In other way, Lilejstrand and Stenström [4] estimated the propulsive forces from the energy consumption. These two methods have been improved by different authors [5],[6],[7]...[8].

More recently, pressure transducers or strain gauges were fixed on the palmar face of the hand in order to evaluate propulsive forces of the hand [9],[10]. Svec [11] improved this method in taking into account the hyrrdodynamic and the hydrostatic pressures. Loetz et al. [12] identified three pressure peaks which occurred at the end of each sculling movement with a maximal value at the end of the inward scull. As mentioned by Barthels [13], high pressures were obtained when pushing backward on a straight line, considering only the drag force. Furthermore, this pressure did not give any information on the direction of the force and on its components [14].

In 1979, Schleihauf [15] tried to determine the lift and drag forces produced by the hand in swimming. He tested different models of the hands in a fluid laboratory in order to determine the lift and drag coefficients under a wide range of flow conditions.

From 3-D kinematic analysis, he calculated velocity, pitch and sweepback angles of the hand to determine lift (L) and drag (D) forces, their resultant (R) and the projection of the resultant on the forward axis (efficient component). Schleihauf [15] noted that the predominance of either the lift or drag forces changed within the stroke. He observed [15],[16] the maximal propulsive force during the final push of the hand for different stroke technique. Maglischo et al [19] noted that the swimmer was able to generate only one or two peaks of propulsive forces during the stroke cycle.

All these studies presented only descriptive results without any question on the relationships between the forces production and the speed of the swimmer, between the forces production and the level of performance. The main question "what is the propulsive force ?" is still open. In other way, the quantification of the force distribution through the different phases of the stroke and its relation to the level of performance have not be studied.

The purpose of this study was to examine time and forces distributions through the different phases of the stroke cycle and the influence of the level of performance on these parameters.

2 Methods

2.1 Subjects
Nine trained competitive swimmers participated in this study. Their general characteristics were presented in table 1.

No significant correlations were observed between the performance and the height or the weight or the age.

Table 1. General characteristics of the studied population (N=9).

Parameter	mean (s.d.)	range
Age (years)	20 (3.16)	8
Height (cm)	184.56 (6.84)	21
Weight (kg)	74.89 (9;19)	24
Performance (%)*	89.88 (7.54)	19.7

*The best time of each swimmer (100m freestyle) was expressed in percentage of the 1988 world record.

2.2 Testing procedures

Each subject swam 4 X 25 m in freestyle at a given speed (1.6 m/s). A rest of 3 minutes was observed between each race to minimize the fatigue. This common speed was chosen in order to examine if the level of performance influenced the times and forces distributions through the phases.

2.3 Data acquisition

During the test, two underwater video cameras (60 Hz) were located in waterproof boxes to get front and side views of the aquatic part of the stroke cycle. Four light emitting diodes were fixed on the hand (fingertip, thumb, pinky and wrist).

2.4 Data treatment

One stroke was digitized frame by frame for each video view. The coordinates in three dimension were obtained for the four points of the hand, the elbow, the shoulder. From the kinematic data and according to Schleihauf's method [15], the lift (L) and drag (D) forces exerted by the hand were determined for each frame.

The resultant (R) of these two forces was calculated. The projection of this resultant force onto the forward axis expressed the efficient component (E.C).

From the side view, four phases were objectively identified from the arm-trunk angle : phase 1: from the hand entry to an arm trunk angle of 30°, phase 2: from 35° to 90°, phase 3: from 90° to 135°, phase 4 : from 135° to the hand exit. Time (ms) and integral values (N.s) of each force (lift, drag, resultant and efficient component) were expressed for the aquatic part of the stroke and each phase. Mean, 1 standard deviation and coefficient of correlation of each parameter with the performance were calculated ($r = 0, 67$ with $p = 0,05$).

3 Results

The times of the different phases (Fig.1) showed a longer first phase (from the hand entry to an arm-trunk angle of 30°), a shorter third phase (90° to 135°) and an equivalent duration for the phases 2 (30° to 90°) and 4 (135° to the hand exit).

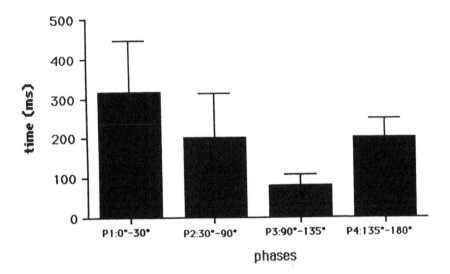

Fig.1. Means and s.d. of the times of the phases.

Although large individual variations were observed for all the phases, only the time of the finish phase presented a significantly negative correlation to the performance (Fig.2). Best performers presented shorter final phase when they swam at the studied speed.

For the aquatic part of the stroke, forces (Fig. 3) indicated higher mean value for the drag than for the lift forces. The population appeared to be more dispersed for the efficient component and the drag forces.

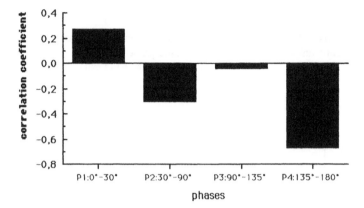

Fig.2.   Coefficients of correlations between the time of the phases and the performance.

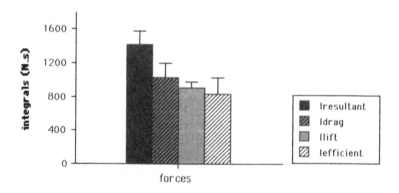

Fig.3.   Means and s.d. of the integrals values of the forces for the aquatic part of the stroke.

No force was significantly correlated to the performance although, the coefficient of correlation was higher for the efficient component and lower for the drag force. Best swimmers tended to present higher efficient component resultant force for the aquatic part of the stroke (Fig.4).

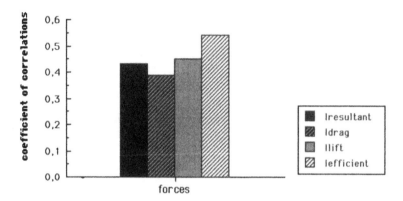

Fig.4. Coefficients of correlations of the integrals forces for the aquatic part of the stroke and the performance.

All the forces (Fig.5) were lower for the first phase and greater for the final phase. Excepted for the final phase, the lift component is lower than the drag component. For all the phases and all the forces, large individual variations were observed.

No significant correlations between forces and level of performance were obtained although the final phase presented higher coefficient. For the common studied speed, best perfomers did not develop higher or lower forces with their hand through all the phases (Fig.6).

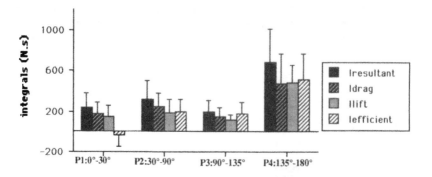

Fig.5.   Means and s.d. of the integrals of the forces for the different phases.

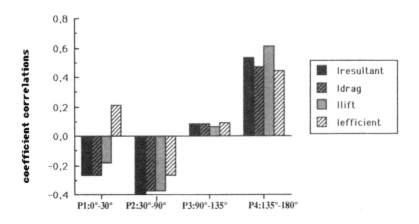

Fig.6.   Coefficients of correlations of the integrals of the forces for each phase and the performance.

4 Discussion

Through the last 20 years, different methods have been used to determine the phases of the stroke. Some authors used the angular velocity of the arm [17], other started from the ratio hand velocity/hip velocity [18].

More recently, Schleihauf [15], and Maglischo [19] identified the phases from typical points reached by the hand in the frontal plane. In other way, Rouard [20], [21] and Hay [22] proposed a phases determination from the arm-trunk angles in the side plane. Although "the division of stroke cycle into phases based upon kinematic parameters" [18] is not yet well standardized, our results confirmed previous findings [20], [21] with a longer first phase and a shorter third phase.

The greater values observed for all the forces during the final phase agreed with Schleihauf observations [23], [16] which noted peak forces at the end of the aquatic part of the stroke for all the models of stroke technique.

The higher production of drag force than lift force through all the phases except for the final phase could be explained by the hand position during this phase. The formula of lift and drag forces $(D = 1/2 \, r \, V^2 \, C_L \, S$ and $L = 1/2 \, r \, V^2 \, C_D \, S$, where r = density of the water, V^2 = hand speed and S = hand surface area,[15]) differed only by the lift and drag coefficients (C_L and C_D). These coefficients were determined from the pitch and sweepback angles of the hand. As a result of theses angles (specially the pitch angle) during the final push, lift coefficient and lift force were higher than drag coefficient and drag force.

The poor correlations between the performance and the different parameters indicated that, for the studied speed, the level of performance did not influence the time and forces distributions except for the final phase. Best performers decreased the time and tended to produce higher hand forces during the end of the push . As a result, they presented more explosive movement for the final part of the stroke. For a given speed, the level of performance did not influence forces and times distributions during the phases of the stroke except for the end of the movement for which best performers appeared to be more explosive.

5 Conclusion

The study of the times and forces distributions through the phases of the stroke showed a longer first phase and greater forces production. during the final phase. Large individual variations were observed for the forces as well as for the times. Poor correlations were obtained between the level of performance and times-forces values for all the phases, except for the final phase. During this phase, best swimmers presented shorter duration and higher forces. A given speed seem to be linked to a given time and forces distributions whatever the level of performance except for the final phase where best performers developed more explosive movements.

In the future, it will be interesting to examine the forces production for the maximal speed of each swimmer in order to determine if the best performers presented higher forces.

6 References

1.   Houssay, R. (1912) Forme, *Puissance et Stabilité des Poissons*, Hermann et Fils, Paris.
2.   Cureton, T.K. (1930) Mechanics and kinesiology of swimming. *Research Quaterly*, 1, pp. 87-121.
3.   Karpovich, P.V. and Pestrecov, K. (1939) Mechanical work and efficiency in swimming crawl and back strokes. Arbeitphysiologie, 10, pp. 504-514.
4.   Lilejstrand, G. and Stenström, N. (1919) Studièn über die physiologie des schwimmens. *Scandinavia Archivia Physiology*, 39, pp. 1-63.
5.   Alley, L. (1952) Analysis of water resistance and propulsion in swimming the crawl stroke. *Research Quaterly*, 23, 3, pp. 253-270.
6.   Costill, D.L. (1966) Use of a swimming ergometer in physiological research. *Research Quaterly*, 37, 4, pp. 564-567.
7.   Faulkner, J.A. (1966) Physiology of swimming. *Research Quaterly*, 37, pp. 41-54.
8.   Magel, J.R. (1970) Propelling force measured during tethered swimming in the four competitve styles. *Research Quaterly*, 41,1, pp. 68-74.
9.   Belokovsky, V. (1971) An analysis of pulling motion in the crawl arm stroke, in *Swimming I* (eds. L.Lewillie, J.P. Clarys), Université Libre de Bruxelles, pp. 217-222.
10.   Van Manen, J.D. and Rijken, H. (1975) Dynamic measurement techniques on swimming bodies at the Netherlands Ship Model Basin, in *Swimming II*, (eds. L. Lewillie and J.P. Clarys), International Series on Sport Sciences, vol 2,University Park Press, Baltimore, pp. 70-79.
11.   Svec, O.J. (1982) Biofeeddback for pulling efficiency. *Swimming Technique*, 19,1, pp. 38-46.
12.   Loetz, C., Reischle, K., Schmitt, G. (1988) The evaluation of highly skilled swimmers via quantitative and qualitative analysis. In *Swimming V*, (eds. B.E.

Ungerechts, K. Wilke and K. Reischle), International Series on Sport Sciences, vol 18, Human Kinetics, Champaign Illinois, pp. 361-367.

13. Barthels, K.M. (1979) The mechanism for body propulsion in swimming, in *Swimming III*, (eds. J. Terauds and E.W. Bedingfield), International Series on Sport Sciences, vol 8, University Park Press, Baltimore, pp.45-54.

14. Schleihauf, R.E. (1986) Swimming skill : a review of basic theory. *Journal of Swimming Research*, 2, 2, pp.11-20.

15. Scheihauf, R.E. (1979) A hydrodynamic analysis of swimming propulsion, in *Swimming III*, (eds. J. Terauds and E.W. Bedingfield), International Series on Sport Sciences, vol 8, University Park Press, Baltimore, pp. 70-109.

16. Scheihauf, R.E., Higgins, J.R., Hinrichs, R., Luedtke, D., Maglischo, C.Maglischo, E.W., Thayer, A. (1988) Propulsive techniques : front crawl stroke, butterfly, backstroke and breaststroke, in *Swimming V*, (eds. B.E. Ungerechts, K. Wilke and K. Reischle), International Series on Sport Sciences, vol 18, Human Kinetics, Champaign Illinois, pp. 53-59.

17. Vaday, M. and Nemessuri, N. (1971) Motor pattern of freestyle swimming, in *Swimming 1* (eds. L.Lewillie, J.P. Clarys), Université Libre de Bruxelles, pp. 167-173.

18. Wiegand, K., Wuensch, D., and Jaehnig, W. (1975) The division of swimming strokes into phases, based upon kinematics parameters, in*Swimming II*, (eds. L. Lewillie and J.P. Clarys), International Series on Sport Sciences, vol 2, University Park Press, Baltimore, pp. 70-79.

19. Maglischo, C.W., Maglischo, E.W., Higgins, J., Hinrichs, R., Luedtke, D., Schleihauf, R.E., Thayer, A. (1988) A biomechanical analysis of the 1984 U.S. Olympic freestyle distance swimmers, in *Swimming V*, (eds. B.E. Ungerechts, K. Wilke and K. Reischle), International Series on Sport Sciences, vol 18, Human Kinetics, Champaign Illinois, pp. 351-360.

20. Rouard A.H. (1987) Etude biomécanique du crawl : évolution des paramètres cinématiques et électromyographiques avec la vitesse. *Thèse* de l'Université J. Fourier, Grenoble, 1, 1987.

21. Rouard, A.H. and Billat, R.P. (1990) Influences of sex and level of performance on freestyle stroke : an electromyographic and kinematic study. *International Journal of Sports Medicine*, vol 11, 2, 150-155.

22. Hay, J. (1988) The status of research on biomechanics of swimming, in*Swkmming V*, (eds. B.E. Ungerechts, K. Wilke and K. Reischle), International Series on Sport Sciences, vol 18, Human Kinetics, Champaign Illinois, pp. 3-14.

23.   Schleihauf, R.E., Gray, L. and DeRose, J. Three dimensional analysis of hand propulsion in the sprint front crawl, in Biomechanics and Medicine in Swimming, (eds. A.P. Hollander, P.A. Huijing and G de Groot), International Series on Sport Sciences, vol 14, Human Kinetics, Champaign Illinois, pp. 173-183.

6 FRONT CRAWL STROKE PHASES: DISCRIMINATING KINEMATIC AND KINETIC PARAMETERS

K.M. MONTEIL*, A.H. ROUARD*, A.B. DUFOUR**,
J.M. CAPPAERT*** and J.P. TROUP***
*Laboratoire de la Performance, C.R.I.S., Lyon France
**Laboratoire d'analyse de données et de biométrie, C.R.I.S., Lyon France
***U.S. Swimming, University of Colorado, Colorado Springs, USA.

Abstract
The purpose of this study was to examine if aquatic phases of the front crawl stroke could be discriminated by kinematic and kinetic parameters. Nine male subjects swam a 400 yards front crawl at their maximal intensity in a flume. Two underwater cameras filmed the subject, in order to obtain three dimensional data from the DLT method. Velocity and forces of the hand, efficiency index, power output and propelling efficiency were calculated. Discriminant analysis was used in order to study the stroke phases for two conditions: before and after exhaustion. Linear correlation coefficients were calculated between the function discriminant and the swimming velocity, in order to point out a performance effect.. Before exhaustion, the combination of efficiency index, propulsive efficiency and component efficient of the resultant discriminated strongly the three phases. The combination of these parameters was not correlated to the swimming velocity. After exhaustion, two combinations were pointed out. The first included efficiency index, component efficient of the resultant and propulsive efficiency. A significant relationships indicated that the best swimmers had the greater values for these parameters during the insweep phase. The second combination was defined by the hand velocity which was not linked to the swimming velocity.
Keywords: Exhaustion, kinematic, kinetic, performance, swimming, phases.

1 Introduction

In swimming, many investigations were conducted on kinematic and kinetic parameters in front crawl stroke. Review of the literature showed that the determination of the aquatic stroke phases was never normalized or validated [1]. All the authors agreed to differentiate two parts in the stroke, the aquatic and the recovery parts. The aquatic part of the stroke, was divided into three or four phases, using different parameters. For the three phases decomposition, the first phase of the stroke could be named catch phase [2] or gliding phase [3] or initial press [4]. The second phase could be defined as the propulsive phase [2] and [3], or as the inward scull [4]. Finally, the last phase could be described as the finish phase [2] and [5] or the outward scull [4]. Some authors have divided the aquatic part of the stroke in 4 phases : catch, pull, push and end push [5], or partitioned as entry, downsweep, insweep and upsweep [6]. Some investigators have taken into account the angle between the arm and the trunk of the body [7]. Others divided the aquatic part of the stroke as introductory, propulsive, transitional and preparatory phases, from the hand and hip velocities [8]. All this various procedures did not allow comparison between authors' findings.

From these previous investigations, it appeared to be interesting to identify kinematic and kinetic parameters discriminating the aquatic phases in front crawl stroke.

2 Methods

2.1 Population
Nine male swimmers, from regional to international level, were volunteer for this study. Their anthropometric characteristics and swimming velocity (Sv) were reported in table 1.

Table 1. Anthropometric and swimming velocity characteristics of the population

	Age(years)	Height (cm)	Weight (kg)	Body fat(%)	Sv (m.s^{-1})
Mean	23.8	184.0	77	9.4	1.62
St. dev.	4.5	5.0	5.8	1.1	0.28
Range	17-30	175-193	70.3-90.7	7.8-10.8	0.95-1.95

For height and weight parameters, population appeared to be homogeneous, whereas age, body fat and swimming velocity, values were rather extended.

2.2 Test and data acquisition
The test took place in a flume (swimming treadmill), where the subject remained on the same place while the water was moving. Each swimmer realized the test in front crawl at his maximal intensity corresponding to a 400 yards. The test was over when the swimmer could not keep the pace and was flowing back in the flume.

During the test, two underwater video cameras filmed the swimmer. The set up was made following Shapiro's considerations [9] in order to obtain valuable three dimensional

(3D) coordinates, from the direct linear transformation method [10]. Aquatic part of the stroke was split into three phases, defined from the motion of the fingertips in the frontal plan: catch (from the hand entry to the more external point), insweep (from the more external to the more internal point) and finish (from the more internal point to the hand exit). Data were collected during the first five seconds (initial condition) and last ones (final condition) of the swimming test. One arm stroke was digitized frame by frame for each condition.

2.3 Data treatment
From the three dimensional video analysis developed by Schleihauf [11], the hand velocity (HV), the resultant hand force (R), its component efficient (RE) defined as its projection on the horizontal axis (motion axis of the swimmer) were calculated. From these parameters, the efficiency index (EFI), the power output (PO) and the propelling efficiency (PE) were computed [12]. The efficiency index (EFI) was defined as the ratio of the resultant hand force on the component efficient (R/RE), in order to quantify the part of the resultant hand force used in the propulsion as a forward motion. The power output, as defined in previous studies [13], [14], [15], was composed by a propulsive part developed to overcome the drag (PD) and a "loss" part used to accelerate water. The propelling efficiency [13], [14], [15] was determined as the ratio of the power developed to overcome the drag (PD) on the power output (PD/PO). These formula were adapted to the flume condition [12]:

2.4 Statistical methods
A discriminant analysis was computed for each condition of the test. This method was used in order to identify the parameters discriminating the aquatic phases of the stroke. Linear correlation coefficients were calculated between the discriminant function and the swimming velocity for each phase and each condition of the test ($r=0.6664$ at $p=0.05$).

3 Results

3.1 Initial condition
Only the first discriminant function ($h^2 = 0.89$) was analyzed (Fig. 1). This function was composed by a combination of the efficiency index, propelling efficiency and component efficient of the resultant hand force.

There was an opposition between the catch phase and the insweep and finish ones. This result indicated that values obtained for the parameters of the combination were greater in the insweep and finish phases than in the catch one. All the swimmers were rather closed from each other : the phases did not differ from one subject to another.

The linear correlation coefficient between the discriminant function of each phase and the swimming velocity values did not show any significant relationships (catch : $r=0.18$; insweep : $r=0.58$; finish : $r=0.11$). In other words, best swimmers did not present higher values for the parameters of the combination.

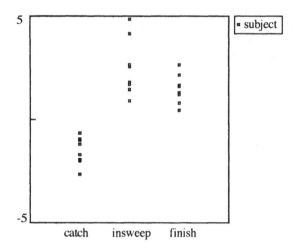

Fig. 1. Representation of the discriminant function of the phases

3.2 Final condition

For the final condition, two discriminant functions were studied. The first one (h^2= 0.96) was composed by the combination of efficiency index, component efficient of the resultant hand force and propulsive efficiency (Fig. 2). This combination was stronger than the one obtained for the initial condition. This could be seen on the representation with the swimmers very grouped together. This result indicated that the phases were strongly differentiated when the swimmer started to be exhausted.

As for the initial condition, this first function opposed the catch phase to the insweep and finish ones. This result underlined that the values of the combined parameters were small for the catch and important for the insweep and the finish phases.

Linear correlation coefficients between this function and swimming velocity indicated an important correlation for the insweep phase (r=0.81 and poor relations for the two others (catch : r=0.04 and finish : r=0.004). This result indicated that greater would be the values of the combined parameters in the insweep phase, higher would be the swimming velocity.

The second discriminant function (h^2= 0.46) was mainly defined by the hand velocity parameter (Fig. 3).

Although this function was less important, it pointed out an important parameter for the analysis of the stroke [16]. This function opposed the insweep phase to the catch and finish ones. The value of the hand velocity was small during the insweep phase and important during the catch and finish ones.

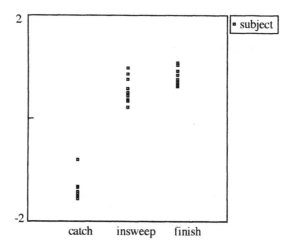

Fig. 2. Representation of the first discriminant function of the phases

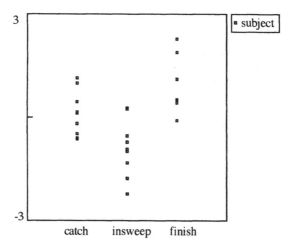

Fig. 3. Representation of the second discriminant function of the phases

No linear correlation coefficient was observed between the second function discriminant for each phase and the swimming velocity. The hand velocity parameter for the different phases did not seem to be linked to the performance.

4 Discussion

For the initial and the final condition, phases were discriminated by the same parameters for each subject, the swimmers being closed from each other. This result pointed out that the discrimination of the phases was not influence by the level of performance of the swimmers. This result was more pronounced, when the swimmer started to be exhausted. Values of the efficiency index, propulsive efficiency and the component efficient of the resultant hand force were very important for the insweep and finish phases. This result indicated that these two phases were very important and linked to the swimming efficiency. The hand velocity appeared to a discriminating parameter only when the subject started to be tired. It decreased during the insweep phase to reach its maximal value during the finish phase. This result confirmed previous findings [17], which obtained a maximal velocity of the hand during the last part of the stroke.

Best swimmers presented greater values of index efficiency, propulsive efficiency and component efficient of the resultant hand force during the insweep phase for the final condition. This result pointed out the importance of this stroke phase for the swimming efficiency, as mentioned by Svec [18].

5. Conclusion

Before exhaustion, the three phases were strongly discriminated by the combination of efficiency index, propulsive efficiency and component efficient of the resultant. No significant relationships between this combination and the swimming velocity was obtained. After exhaustion, two combinations emerged. The first included efficiency index, component efficient of the resultant and propulsive efficiency. A significant relationships indicated that the best swimmers had the greater values for these parameters during the insweep phase. The second combination was defined by the hand velocity which was not related to the performance.

6 References

1.   Persyn, U., Daly, D.J., Thewissen, M. and Vervaecke, H. (1976) The synchronization problem in swimming. *Hermès* (Leuven), X, pp. 409-431.
2.   Counsilman, J.E. (1968) *The science of swimming*, Prentice Hall, Inc, Englewood cliffs, N.J.
3.   Vaday, M. and Nemessuri, M. (1971) Motor pattern of freestyle swimming. *Biomechanics of Swimming*, (ed. L. Lewillie and J.P. Clarys), Brussels: Université Libre de Bruxelles, pp. 167-173.
4.   Hay, J.G. (1985) Swimming. *The Biomechanics of Sports Techniques*, Prentice-Hall, Inc., Englewood Cliffs, N.J.

5. Haljand R. (1985) Une nouvelle approche scientifique de l'analyse des nages. Doc FFN. Traduction M. Knoop, pp.1-32.

6. Maglischo, C.W., Maglischo, E.W., Sharp, R.L., Zier, D.J. and Katz, A. (1984) Tethered and non tethered crawl swimming. *Sports Biomechanics*, (ed. J. Terauds, K. Barthels, E. Kreighbaum, R. Mannand J. Crakes), Del Mar: Research center for sports, pp. 163-176.

7. Rouard, A.H. (1987) Etude biomécanique du crawl: évolution des paramètres cinématiques et électromyographiques avec la vitesse. Thèse de doctorat, Université Grenoble I.

8. Wiegand, K., Wuensch, D. and Jaehnig, W. (1975) The division of swimming strokes into phases, based upon kinematic parameters. *Swimming II*, (ed. L. Lewillie and J.P. Clarys), Baltimore: University Park Press, pp. 161-166.

9. Shapiro, R. (1978) Direct Linear Transformation method for three-dimensional cinematography. *Research Quarterly*, 49, pp. 197-205.

10. Abdel-Azziz, Y.I. and Karara, H.M. (1971) Direct Linear Transformation from comparator coordinates into,object space coordinates in close-range photogrammetry. *ASP Symposium on Close-Range Photogrammetry*, American Society of Photogrammetry, Falls Church, pp.1-18.

11. Schleihauf, R.E. (1979) A hydrodynamic analysis of swimming propulsion. *Swimming III*, (ed. J. Terauds and E.W. Bedeingfield), 8, Baltimore: University Park Press, pp.70-109.

12. Cappaert, J.M., Franciosi, P., Langhns, G. and Troup, J.P. (1990) Indirect calculation of mechanical and propelling efficiency during freestyle swimming. *Abstracts of the Sixth International Symposium on Biomechanics and Medicine in Swimming*, Liverpool Polytechnic, Liverpool.

13. Huijing, P.A., Hollander, A.P. and Groot, G. de (1983) Efficiency and specificity of training in swimming: an editorial. *Biomechanics and Medicine in Swimming*, (ed. A.P. Hollander, P.A. Huijing and G. de Groot)14, Champaign: Human Kinetics Publishers Inc., pp. 1-6.

14. Toussaint, H.M., Helm, F.C.T. van der, Elzerman, J.R., Hollander, A.P., Groot, G. de and Ingen Schenau, C.J. van (1983) A power balance applied to swimming. *Biomechanics and Medi cine in Swimming*, (ed. A.P. Hollander, P.A. Huijing and G. de Groot)14, Champaign: Human Kinetics Publishers Inc., pp. 165-172.

15. Toussaint, H.M. (1988) Mechanics and energetics of swimming. Ph. D. Thesis, Rodopi, Amsterdam, 1988.

16. Rackham, G.W. (1975) Analysis of arm propulsion in swimming. *Swimming II*, (ed. L. Lewillie and J.P. Clarys), Baltimore: University Park Press, pp. 174-179.

17. Welch, J.H. (1974) A kinematic analysis of world-class crawl stroke swimmers. *Biomechanics iV* (ed. R.C. Nelson and C.A. Morehouse), Baltimore: University Park Press, pp. 217-222.

18. Svec, O.J. (1982) Biofeedback of pulling efficiency. *Swimming technique*, 19, pp. 38-46.

7 RELATIONSHIPS BETWEEN THE THREE COORDINATES OF THE UPPER LIMB JOINTS WITH SWIMMING VELOCITY

V.J. DESCHODT, A.H. ROUARD and K.M. MONTEIL
Laboratoire de la Performance, C.R.I.S., U.F.R.A.P.S. Lyon
France

Abstract
The aim of the study was to examine the relationships between the movements,of the upper limb joints, in the three dimensions. 44 swimmers were filmed during the 100m freestyle races of the national Championships, using two videocameras. According to Schleihauf 's method, the coordinates of the wrist, the elbow and the shoulder were obtained. In the horizontal axis, the wrist presented a sinusoïdal path. This joint moved forward, then backward in the middle of the time of the stroke, and forward again before the exit. The elbow had a sinusoïdal path but flater than the wrist.The shoulder had a linear displacement. In the lateral axis, the wrist have a tendancy to move outsweep in the middle part of the stroke, contrary to the elbow which moved insweep. During all the stroke, the shoulder had an inside displacement. For the vertical axis, all the joints moved down. The relationships between each dimension showed that the hip velocity was related to the horizontal and vertical displacements of the joints and not linked to lateral movements.
Keywords :freestyle, displacements, upper limb, three dimensions.

1 Introduction

Brown and Counsilman [1] have shown the sinusoïdal aquatic trajectory of the hand. Using underwater videos, Schleihauf [2] confirmed that the hand movement was not only in the forward-backward direction, but presented also lateral and vertical movements. Webb [3] have observed that the fish moved its tails inside with an angle in regard to the axis of the water, resulting in a backward and sideways movement of the water which allowed to the body to moved forward through the water. The same action could be used by the swimmer who moved his hands outwards and inswards from the longitudinal axis of the body, defined as sculling movements. Swimmers did not push the water directly backward, but should use sculling motions of their hands and feet to propel them forward [1,2]. This sculling movement of the hand would allow to the swimmer to increase his propulsive efficiency in pushing a lot of water on a short distance". Barthels [4] have noted that this sculling movement allowed to the hand to stay fixed, and to the shoulder to overcross forward the hand and the elbow.

Studying high level swimmers, Schleihauf [2] described three different patterns of aquatic movement of the hand, in three dimensions.

The aim of our study was to examine the relationships between each dimension of the movement for the shoulder, elbow and hand and their contribution to the hip velocity .

2 Protocol and measurements

2.1 Protocol
44 swimmers have been studied during the 100 m freestyle races of the National Championships. Their characteristics datas were reported in the table 1

Table 1: Characteristics datas of the population (N=44)

Parameters	Average	s.d.	Range
Weight (kg)	78.94	15.02	27.2
Height (cm)	1.847	0.11	0.16
Age (years)	21.4	6.29	11
Performance in 100m races (s)	51.02	4.42	7.18

2.2 Measurements
Two video camecorders (30 Hz) have been used to film the swimmers on 15 meters, at the extremity of the length of the swimming pool, before the turn. They were synchronized and fixed in underwater boxes (60 cm depth) with an angle to 90° between themselves.

Each view was digitized frame by frame, according to Schleihauf [2]. From this digitalisation, 2 Dimensions coordinates were obtained for the wrist, the elbow and the shoulder joints during the cycle. One cycle was defined by the hand entry to the hand exit. The two coordinates have been computed to give the 3 Dimensions coordinates : (x): horizontal, (y): lateral and (z): vertical dimensions.

3 Results

3.1 Mean trajectory of the joints :
For each frame, each joint and each dimension, we have calculated the mean (s.d) coordinate for the 44 subjects to get the mean trajectory of the studied population.

For the horizontal displacement (Fig.1), the wrist presented a sinusoïdal path. It did not stay fixed on the aquatic part of the stroke. It moved first forward up to 29.63 % of the total time of the cycle, backward up to 77.77 % and forward to the end of the cycle. The amplitude of the backward motion of the wrist was 0.80 m. This joint was again at the coordinate of the initial entry point above the middle part of the stroke (55.55 %). During this phase of the movement, the population appeared very dispersed. The elbow had a similar sinusoïdal path but flater than the wrist trajectory. The elbow slipped less backward, than the wrist (0.20 m). As a result, this joint did not come back to the coordinate of the point entry. In regard to the standard deviation, the population was more homogeneous for the elbow trajectory than for the wrist one. The shoulder joint had a linear and regular displacement during the stroke. The standard deviation have a tendancy to increase with the displacement reflecting a dispersion of the population at the end of the stroke cycle.

For the vertical axis, the wrist (Fig.2) was oriented down up to 55.55 % of the total time cycle. The maximal depth was 0.78 m. After this maximal point, the wrist moved up until the hand exit. The duration of the first part of the down movement was longer than the up one. The standard deviation were more important during the end of the first part. The elbow would have the same trajectory of the wrist with a lower depth (0.45 m). Contrary to the two first joints, the shoulder was more fixed on the vertical axis. Its maximal depth was 0.15 m. In regard to the large standard deviation, some swimmers presented very large vertical variations of the shoulder.

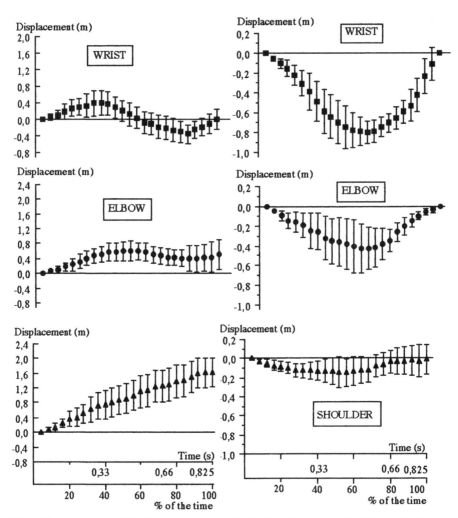

Fig.1. Mean trajectory (s.d.) of the wrist, elbow and shloulder joints on the horizontal axis

Fig 2. Mean trajectory (s.d.) of the wrist, elbow and shoulder on the vertical axis (oz)

For the lateral dimension, the wrist (Fig.3) seemed stay in the same position up to 29.63 % of the total time of the cycle, i.e. little right-left movements were observed. After this time, the hand presented outsweep trajectory up to 62.96 % of the total time of the cycle, and finish the stroke with an insweep movement. The large standard deviations showed that the swimmers presented very different lateral deviations of the wrist, especially during the insweep phase. For the elbow joint, lateral variations in the trajectories occured at the same time than the wrist (29.63 % and 62.96 % of the total time of the stroke). When the wrist had an insweep displacement, the elbow presented an outside movement. The population was very heterogeneous for the lateral trajectory of the elbow. Through all the aquatic cycle, the shoulder had an inside displacement. As for the other joints, the lateral trajectory of the shoulder presented large individual variations.

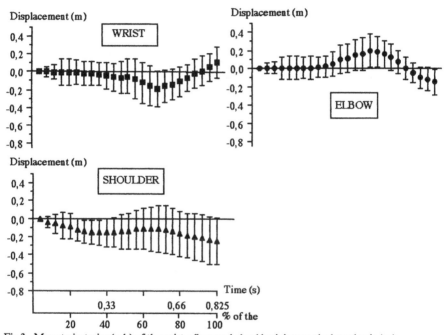

Fig.3. Mean trajectories (s.d.) of the wrist, elbow and shoulder joints on the lateral axis (oy)

3.2 Amplitude of the joints :

For each joint and each dimension, we have calculated the mean range of the movement (Fig. 4). The range of the horizontal displacement decreased from the proximal joint (shoulder) to the distal one (hand). An opposite tendancy was observed for the vertical movement. Wrist presented greater vertical than horizontal displacements. Results were opposite for the shoulder. For the lateral movements, elbow and shoulder joints showed the same ranges, which were less important than the wrist.

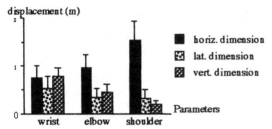

Figure 4. Descriptive analysis of the upper limb joints in the three dimensions.

3.3 Relationships between each dimension :

The relations between the parameters themselves and with the hip velocity was studied with a principal component analysis. The representation of this statistic test was the correlation cercle (Fig.5). The axis 1 was defined by the hip velocity in the horizontal dimension (1), and the axis 2 by the length of the upper limb joint in the lateral dimension (6 to 9). Two groups of parameters can be observed. The first group was constitued by the hip velocity (1) and the horizontal (No2 to 5) and vertical (No10 to 13) displacements of the wrist, elbow and shoulder. The closed position of theses parameters reflected the strong relationships of the hip velocity wiht the horizontal and vertical movements of the upper limb. In other words, to increase the hip velocity, swimmers would increase the horizontal and vertical amplitudes of the upper limb joints movements. The second group (No6 to 9) showed that the lateral movements did not contribued to the hip velocity. Moreover, they were not dependant of the vertical and horizontal displacements of the joint.

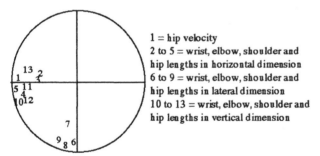

1 = hip velocity
2 to 5 = wrist, elbow, shoulder and hip lengths in horizontal dimension
6 to 9 = wrist, elbow, shoulder and hip lengths in lateral dimension
10 to 13 = wrist, elbow, shoulder and hip lengths in vertical dimension

Fig.5. Correlation cercle of upper limb lengths in the three dimensions and hip velocity.

4 Comments

Contrary to previous studies [4], [5], [6], our results showed that the wrist was not fixed during the aquatic stroke in freestyle. The wrist had a sinusoïdal path in the antero-posterior axis.. This joint was gone out the water on the same point than the entry point. It was going forward at the beginning of the cycle according [2], [7], [8] then backward behind the entry point, before to move forward again at the end of the stroke. This forward displacement could result from the movement of the other arm and/or the legs actions. The elbow had a sinusoïdal displacement, but flater than the wrist. The shoulder had a constant displacement in this axis. In the same way, Reischle [11] have observed that a regular hip displacement was very linked to the performance. The sweep of the hand and of the elbow could allow to the shoulder and so to the body to have this regular progression. In the lateral axis, the wrist presented outsweep displacement, contrary to the elbow what had an insidedisplacement during the middle part of the stroke. In the vertical axis, all the joints were oriented first down during the first part of the cycle, then they moved up until the exit. The standard deviation were more important during the end of the first part for all the joints. The most important displacement have been reported in the horizontal dimension [9], [2], [10]. The hand had more important variations in the lateral and vertical dimensions than the other joints. Maglischo [10] described swimmers who tended to favor either lateral or vertical strocking motions. Our study have shown that the range in the horizontal and vertical dimension were positively and significatly linked to the hip velocity. More the swimmer would have greater horizontal and vertical sweeps, more the hip velocity would be important. Any relation between the lateral variation and the body velocity have been observed, contrary to other studies [15], [1], who suggested that the hand of elite swimmers should follow a path, described as either "a bottom-heavy S", or contrary to Rackham [3], who noted the relation between the deviation in the three dimensions and the body velocity.

5 Conclusion :

The study of the trajectories in three dimensions of the joints of the upper limb movements pointed out that the hand was not fixed on the antero-posterieur axis contrary as mentionned by different authors. Although the hand exit at the same point of the entry, its moves forward during the first part of the stroke and backward up to the end of the stroke. As for the wrist, the elbow presented a flater sinusoidal trajectory although the shoulder had a linear displacement. From the lateral point of view, the wrist moved outside during the middle part of the stroke when the elbow presented an opposite inside movement. The shoulder presented an inside trajectory during all the stroke. On the vertical axis, the three joints moved down than up, shoulder being more fixed for this dimension. The hip velocity appeared to be related to the combination of vertical and horizontal movements of the joints and not to the lateral ones contrary as observed in previous studies.

6 References

1. Brown, R.M., Counsilman, J.E. (1971) The role of lift in propelling the swimmer. *J.M. Cooper (ed), Proceedings of the CIC Symposium on Biomechanics*, pp. 179-188, Indiana University.
2. Schleihauf, R.E. (1979) A hydrodynamic analysis of swimming propulsion. *J. Teraud and E.W. Bedingfield (eds), Swimming III, International Series on Sport Sciences*, Vol. 8, pp. 70-109, University Park Press, Baltimore.
3. Webb, P.W., (1984) Fish swimming, form and function. *Scientific Review*, pp58.
4. Barthels, K.M. (1977) Analysing Swimming Performance: General considerations. *Swimming Technique*, Vol. 14, No.2.pp.51-52.
5. Adams, T.M. (1981) Basic biomechanics for swimming. *Swimming Technique*, Nov.81-Jan.82, pp.41-45.
6. O'Shea, P. (1991) The 50-meter freestyle sprint. *National Strength and Conditioning Association Journal*, Vol.13, No. 5.pp.6-11.
7   Welch, J. (1981) Swimming with accessories: a filmed case study. *Swimming Technique*, Feb.-April, pp.18-19.

8. Counsilman, J.E. (1981) Hand speed and acceleration. *Swimming Technique*, Vol. 18, No. 1, pp. 22-26.
9. Wiegand, K., Wuensch, D., Jaehnig, W. (1975) The division of swimming strokes into phases, based upon kinematic parameters. *L. Lewillie and J.P. Clarys (eds), Swimming II, International Series on Sport Sciences*, Vol. 2, pp. 161-166, University Park Press, Baltimore.
10. Maglischo, C.W., Maglischo, E.W., Higgins, J., Hinricks, R., Luedtke, D., Schleihauf, R.E., Thayer, A. (1986) A biomechanical analysis of the 1984 U.S. Olympic Swimming Team: the distance freestylers. *Journal of Swimming Research*, Vol. 2, No. 3, pp. 12-16.
11. Reischle, K. (1979) Kinematic investigation of movement patterns in swimming with photooptical methods. *Terauds J. and bedingfield E.W. (eds), Swimming III*, pp.127-136, International Symposium of Biomechanics in Swimming, University of Alberta.
12. Kornecki, S. and Bober, T. (1978) Extreme velocities of swimming cycle as a technique criterion. *B. Erikson and B. Furberg (eds), Swimming Medicine IV*, pp.402-407, University Park Press, Baltimore.
13. Toussaint, H.M., Van der Helm, F.C., Elzerman, J.R., Hollander, A.P., Van Ingen Schenau, G.J. (1983) A power balance applied to swimming. *A.P. Hollander, P.A. Huijing, G. de Groot (eds), Biomechanics and Medicine in Swimming, International Series on Sport Sciences*, Vol. 14, pp.165-172, Human kinetics Publishers, Inc., Champaign, Illinois.
14. Nigg, B.M. (1983) Selected methodology in biomechanics with respect to swimming. *A.P. Hollander, P.A. Huijing, G. de Groot (eds), Biomechanics and Medicine in Swimming, International Series on Sport Sciences*, Vol. 14, pp.72-80, Human kinetics Publishers, Inc., Champaign, Illinois.
15. Counsilman, J.E. (1969) The role of Sculling Movements in the arm pull. *Swimming World*, Vol.10, No.12.pp.6-7-43.

8 EFFECT OF BODY ROLL ON HAND VELOCITY IN FREESTYLE SWIMMING

C.J. PAYTON
Division of Sport Science, The Manchester Metropolitan University, Alsager, UK

D.R. MULLINEAUX
School of Human Studies, University of Teesside, Middlesborough, UK

Abstract

A mathematical model was developed [1] to evaluate the contribution of body roll to medial-lateral (v_X) and vertical (v_Z) hand velocities in freestyle swimming. The right arm was modelled as two rigid segments joined at the elbow to enable flexion and extension. The arm was linked to a rigid trunk with a joint capable of shoulder extension and abduction/adduction.

Simulations were performed for pull times (t_{PULL}) from 0.7 s to 1.1 s and maximum body rolls (θ_{MAX}) from 50° to 70° with a straight arm, and with the elbow flexing through 90°. For a simulation involving elbow flexion ($t_{PULL} = 0.7$ s, $\theta_{MAX} = 60°$), mean values for v_X and v_Z were 1.86 m/s and 2.24 m/s respectively. These values were 24% and 22% less, respectively, than those obtained from an equivalent simulation performed with a straight arm. These reduced velocities were due to the elbow flexion: 1) reducing the hand's radii of rotation, and 2) creating a hand velocity component which opposed that resulting from body roll.

It was concluded that body roll makes a substantial contribution to medial-lateral and vertical hand velocities in freestyle swimming and may therefore play an important role in the generation of propulsive lift forces.

Keywords: Body roll, freestyle swimming, hand velocity, modelling.

1 Introduction

When freestyle swimmers scull their hands vertically and medial-laterally, a forwards acting lift force is generated. It has been suggested that these lift forces can make a significant contribution to propulsion [2]. Since lift forces are proportional to the square of the hand speed, forwardly directed (propulsive) lift forces will be a function of the vertical and medial-lateral hand velocities produced by the swimmer.

Little attempt has been made to identify the body movements responsible for generating medial-lateral and vertical hand velocities in the freestyle. Although it seems logical that elbow flexion and shoulder adduction should make a contribution to hand velocity, a recent study [1] questioned the role played by elbow and shoulder movements. Using a mathematical model the authors demonstrated that medial deviations of the hand to the midline of the trunk could be achieved entirely with body roll, without the need for elbow flexion or shoulder adduction. It was also found that the amount of body roll required to sweep the hand to the midline was only 19°-34°. As this was well below the mean maximum body roll value of 60.8° exhibited by ten male university swimmers [3], it was suggested that swimmers may move their arms laterally relative to the trunk in order to avoid pulling the hand too far across the midline of the trunk.

As body roll appears to influence medial-lateral displacement of the hand relative to the water, it must also contribute to medial-lateral hand velocity. It then follows that body roll may assist in the generation of propulsive lift forces in freestyle swimming. The aim of this study was to determine the effect of body roll on medial-lateral and vertical hand velocities during the pull phase in freestyle swimming.

2 Methods

A previous three-dimensional model [1] was modified for this study. The right arm was modelled as two rigid segments hinged at the elbow (E) to enable flexion and extension. The arm was linked to a rigid trunk with a joint (S) capable of shoulder extension and shoulder abduction/adduction (Figure 1).

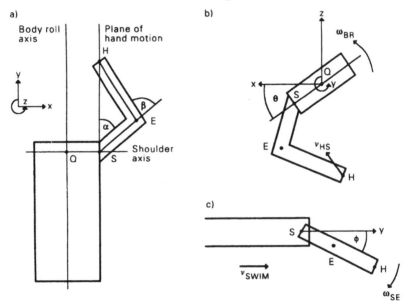

Figure 1. Model viewed in frontal plane (a), transverse plane (b) and sagittal plane (c).

The trunk was free to rotate about its long axis - the *body roll axis*. The hand (H) was constrained to move in the plane located through joint S and normal to the *shoulder axis* - the line connecting the two shoulder joints. The shoulder abduction angle (α) was therefore a function of the elbow angle (β) to ensure the hand remained in this plane - the *plane of hand motion*.

The half shoulder width (l_{QS}), upper arm length (l_{SE}) and forearm plus hand length (l_{EH}) were assigned values of 0.25 m, 0.35 m and 0.5 m respectively, based on reported anthropometric data on competitive swimmers [3].

Simulations were run for fast (0.7 s), medium (0.9 s) and slow (1.1 s) pull times. Within this time:

1. The trunk rotated from a neutral position ($\theta = 0°$) to a pre-selected maximum body roll angle (θ_{MAX}) of either 50°, 60° or 70°, and back to the neutral position.
2. The shoulder extended through 180° from a position of full flexion ($\phi = 0°$).
3. The elbow flexed through 90° from an extended position ($\beta = 0°$) and then fully extended again.

The body roll and elbow flexion angular velocities (ω_{BR} and ω_{β} respectively) were modelled as sine functions such that they were zero at the start, midpoint ($t_{PULL}/2$) and end of each simulation. The shoulder extension angular velocity (ω_{SE}) was held constant in each simulation. The effect of ω_{BR} on hand velocity was dependent on the perpendicular vector from the hand to the body roll axis (l_{YH}). Similarly, the effect of ω_{SE} on hand velocity was a function of the shoulder to hand vector (l_{SH}).

The elbow flexion angular velocity, coupled with the shoulder abduction angular velocity (ω_{α}), produces a hand velocity component (v_{HS}) directed toward the shoulder (Figure 1b). The effect of ω_{α} and ω_{β} on v_{HS} was determined by the lengths of the two arm segments (l_{SE} and l_{EH}).

The equations used to compute the medial-lateral (v_X), superior-inferior (v_Y) and vertical (v_Z) components of the hand velocity, relative to a pool-fixed Cartesian reference frame (Figure 1a), are presented in Table 1.

Table 1. Equations for computing the Cartesian components of the hand velocity.

Body roll	Shoulder extension	Elbow flexion	
$v_X = \omega_{BR} \cdot l_{YH} \cdot \sin \delta$	$+ \, \omega_{SE} \cdot l_{SH} \cdot \cos \phi \cdot \sin \theta$	$+ \, v_{HS} \cdot \sin \phi \cdot \sin \theta$	(1)
$v_Y =$	$\omega_{SE} \cdot l_{SH} \cdot \sin \phi$	$+ \, v_{HS} \cdot \cos \phi \cdot \cos \theta \; + \; v_{SWIM}$	(2)
$v_Z = \omega_{BR} \cdot l_{YH} \cdot \cos \delta$	$+ \, \omega_{SE} \cdot l_{SH} \cdot \cos \phi \cdot \cos \theta$	$+ \, v_{HS} \cdot \sin \phi \cdot \cos \theta$	(3)

where δ is the angle vector l_{YH} makes to the vertical.

3 Results

Table 2 presents the mean hand velocity components from a representative simulation performed without elbow flexion ($\theta_{MAX} = 60°$, $t_{PULL} = 0.7$ s). Table 3 presents mean hand velocity components from an equivalent simulation performed with the elbow flexing through 90°. Mean hand velocity components were defined as the mean absolute value (magnitude) of the hand velocity component from t = 0 to t$_{PULL}$.

The contributions made by body roll, shoulder extension and elbow flexion to the mean hand velocity components are also shown in Tables 2 and 3. The contributions made by elbow flexion to v_X and v_Z have been assigned a negative value. This indicates that elbow flexion served to reduce the mean value of these two velocity components. Swimming velocity (v_{SWIM}) was assumed to remain constant within each simulation and was given an arbitrary value of 1.8 m/s. This value has been included in the calculation of the mean superior-inferior (v_Y) hand velocity values.

Table 2. Mean hand velocity components from a simulation with 60° of body roll, a pull time of 0.7 s, a swim velocity of 1.8 m/s and no elbow flexion.

	Body roll contribution (m/s)	Shoulder ext. contribution (m/s)	Mean velocity (m/s)
v_X	1.67	0.78	2.45
v_Y	-	2.43	0.63
v_Z	0.71	2.17	2.88

Table 3. Mean hand velocity components from a simulation with 60° of body roll, a pull time of 0.7 s, a swim velocity of 1.8 m/s and the elbow flexing through 90°.

	Body roll contribution (m/s)	Shoulder ext. contribution (m/s)	Elbow flexion contribution (m/s)	Mean velocity (m/s)
v_X	1.52	0.68	-0.35	1.85
v_Y	-	2.05	0.30	0.55
v_Z	0.56	2.07	-0.39	2.24

4 Discussion

The effect of body roll on the medial-lateral (v_X), superior-inferior (v_Y) and vertical (v_Z) hand velocities are described by equations 1, 2 and 3 respectively. The equations reveal that body roll angular velocity has a direct influence on medial-lateral and vertical hand velocities but has no effect on the superior-inferior component.

When the body rolls through 60° in 0.35 s (t$_{PULL}$/2) with a fully extended arm, the mean medial-lateral and vertical hand velocities produced are 2.45 m/s and 2.88 m/s respectively (Table 2). For identical body roll conditions, but with the elbow flexing through 90°, the mean medial-lateral hand velocity is reduced by 24% to 1.85 m/s. There is also a 22% reduction in the mean vertical hand velocity to 2.24 m/s resulting from elbow flexion. Although it has previously been suggested [4] that elbow flexion makes a positive contribution to medial-lateral and vertical hand velocities, these results do not support this view.

Elbow flexion reduces the mean medial-lateral and vertical hand velocities in two ways. Firstly, elbow flexion reduces the shoulder to hand distance l_{SH}. Consequently, for any given shoulder extension angle ϕ, the perpendicular distance from the hand to the body roll axis l_{YH} is also reduced. These shortened radii reduce the body roll and shoulder extension contributions to the mean medial-lateral and vertical velocities (Table 3). Secondly, elbow flexion, coupled with shoulder abduction, produces a hand velocity component (v_{HS}) directed toward the shoulder (Figure 1b). The medial-lateral and vertical components of v_{HS} will always oppose the direction of the body roll and shoulder extension contributions to hand velocity.

Of the 24% reduction in medial-lateral hand velocity caused by elbow flexion, 10% is attributable to the shortening of l_{SH} and l_{YH}. The remaining 14% reduction is due to the direction of the medial-lateral component of v_{HS}. Similarly, of the 22% decrease in vertical hand velocity, 8% results from the shortened radii with the vertical component of v_{HS} accounting for the remaining 14%.

In addition to directly contributing to hand velocity ($\omega_{BR} \wedge l_{YH}$), body roll also influences the medial-lateral and vertical velocicities produced by shoulder extension. Equation 1 shows that once body roll has commenced ($\theta \neq 0$), shoulder extension makes a contribution to medial-lateral hand velocity. For a given shoulder extension angle ϕ, the greater the body roll, the greater is the contribution. The inverse is true for vertical hand velocity (Equation 3), as body roll increases (for a given ϕ) the magnitude of this component decreases.

The validity of the model presented in this paper has not yet been established. The results must therefore only be considered as tentative indications of how body roll affects hand velocity in the freestyle. Nevertheless, body roll may make a substantial contribution to medial-lateral and vertical hand velocities in freestyle swimming and therefore play an important role in the generation of propulsive lift forces.

5 References

1. Hay, J.G., Liu, Q., and Andrews, J.G. (1993) Body roll and handpath in freestyle swimming: a computer simulation study. *Journal of Applied Biomechanics*, Vol. 9, No. 3. pp. 227-237.
2. Schleihauf, R.E., Gray, L., and DeRose, J. (1983) Three-dimensional analysis of hand propulsion in the sprint front crawl stroke, in *Biomechanics and Medicine in Swimming,* (eds. A.P. Hollander, P.A. Huijing and G. de Groot), Human Kinetics, Champaign, pp. 173-183.
3. Liu, Q., Hay, J.G., and Andrews, J.G. (1993) Body roll and handpath in freestyle swimming: an experimental study. *Journal of Applied Biomechanics*, Vol. 9, No. 3. pp. 238-253.
4. Barthels, K.M. (1979) The mechanism for body propulsion in swimming, in *Swimming III*, (eds. J. Terauds and E.W. Bedingfield), University Park Press, Baltimore, pp. 45-54.

9 BREASTSTROKE TECHNIQUE VARIATIONS AMONG NEW ZEALAND PAN PACIFIC SQUAD SWIMMERS

R.H. SANDERS
School of Physical Education
University of Otago, Dunedin, New Zealand

Abstract
The purpose of this study was to quantitatively analyse New Zealand's most elite breaststroke swimmers to learn more about the techniques being used and their variability among swimmers of Pan Pacific qualifying standard. Three male and three female New Zealand Pan Pacific Squad members who race in breaststroke and/or individual medley were requested to swim breaststroke at race pace. Two PAL video cameras simultaneously recorded the above and below water views from a position perpendicular to the line of travel of each swimmer. Paths of the shoulders, hips, knees, ankles, feet, center of mass, and trunk and thigh angles were obtained from the digitised records. Pull, kick, glide, and deadspace times, stroke length and stroke frequency, and center of mass velocity were calculated. Large differences among the swimmers were found in all of these variables and swimmers had their own characteristic profiles. In particular, there were large variations in stroke frequencies and stroke lengths, relative durations of the phases, and the amplitudes of vertical undulations of the joint centers and centers of mass. It was concluded that among elite New Zealand breaststrokers there was considerable variability in techniques.
Keywords: Breaststroke, swimming, technique, wave action.

1 Introduction

In recent years many competitive swimmers have changed their breaststroke techniques markedly following the introduction of a new style in which a 'wave action' of the body is utilised [1]. This technique is otherwise known as the 'undulating breaststroke technique'. The main feature that distinguishes the wave action from conventional breaststroke (otherwise termed 'flat' breaststroke) is the high shoulder action and the forward lunge of the upper body above the water during the period between the pull and kick. There are also differences in the amount of undulation of the body parts, and the angles of the body segments [2].

While the wave action technique appears to suit some swimmers and improves their times it has not been universally adopted. Some swimmers have retained the conventional flat style and there appears to be a continuum between the two styles. The purpose of this study was to quantitatively analyse New Zealand's most elite breaststroke swimmers to learn more about the techniques being used and the variability among successful breaststroke swimmers.

2 Method

Three male (M1, M2, M3) and three female (F1, F2, F3) New Zealand Pan Pacific Squad members who race in breaststroke and/or individual medley participated in this study. Swimmers were marked with black tape at points in line with the shoulder, elbow, wrist, hip, knee, and ankle axes of rotation. Scale lines with markers at 50 cm intervals were stretched tightly above and below the line of motion of the swimmers. These were placed seven lanes away from the cameras.

The swimmers were requested to swim at race pace through the recording area. One Panasonic M40 standard PAL video camera and one Panasonic M7 standard PAL video camera simultaneously recorded the above and below water views of the swimmers from the side at 50 fields per second. The cameras were panned to maximise image size.

The above and below water views were digitised on a PEAK Performance 2D digitising system. Bilateral symmetry was assumed and only the camera side of the body was digitised to define an eight segment body model comprising head and neck, trunk, arms, forearms, hands, thighs, shanks, and feet. The raw digitised points from the above and below views were then scaled, aligned using the known positions of points digitised from the scale lines, and combined to produce coordinates for the whole body using a FORTRAN program. Center of mass (CM) was determined by applying the anthropometric data of Dempster [3].

Data corresponding to one stroke cycle, defined as the period from the instant of shoulder entry to the next, were then analysed. Cycles in which the camera axes were close to perpendicular to the swimming direction were selected for analysis.

The variables quantified in this study were stroke length, stroke frequency, the durations of the kick, glide, pull, and deadspace phases of the stroke cycle, CM velocity in the swimming direction (horizontal), range of vertex, shoulder, hip, and CM vertical motion, and trunk and thigh angles.

3 Results

3.1 Vertex, shoulder, hip, and CM undulation
Table 1 shows the range of vertical motion of the vertex, shoulder, hip, and CM. On the basis of these results M1, M2, and F1 were regarded as being predominantly 'wave action' swimmers and F2, F3, and M3 were regarded as 'conventional' or 'flat' breaststrokers.

Table 1. Vertical Undulations

Swimmer	Vertex (cm)	Shoulder (cm)	Hip (cm)	CM (cm)
M1	64	45	13	23
M2	49	32	17	15
M3	46	32	11	10
F1	64	50	15	25
F2	46	21	14	8
F3	43	25	12	10

Vertical undulations of the vertex ranged from 43 cm (F3) to 64 cm (F1 and M1). Vertical undulations of the shoulder ranged from 21 cm (F2) to 50 cm (F1). The undulations of M1 (45 cm) and F1 (50 cm) were comparable to those of Mike Barrowman (44 cm) [4]. Hip undulations ranged from 11 cm (F3) to 17 cm (M2). These were less than those of Mike Barrowman (21 cm). All subjects had large vertex and shoulder undulations compared to the hip undulations. All squad members had vertex and shoulder undulations that were almost opposite in phase to the hip undulations. That is, when the shoulders were at their highest point the hips were near their lowest. The flat breaststroke swimmers (M3, F2, and F3) had small CM undulations (10 cm, 8 cm, and 10 cm respectively) while M1 (23 cm), M2 (15 cm) and F1 (25 cm) had comparatively large CM undulations.

3.2 Stroke frequency, stroke length, and average CM horizontal velocity
Table 2 shows stroke frequency, stroke length (the distance travelled by the CM during the cycle) and the average CM horizontal velocity for the stroke cycle.

Average CM velocity ranged from 1.01 m/s (F2) to 1.26 m/s (M2). These were below the swimmers' usual race pace velocities. It should be borne in mind that although the New Zealand squad members were requested to swim at race pace there was not the pressure of competition and this may have influenced the results.

Stroke frequencies ranged from 0.54 cycles/s (F1) to 0.98 cycles/s (F3). For both the males and females the flat breaststroke swimmers had the greatest stroke frequencies. Stroke lengths ranged from 1.22 m (F3) to 2.13 m (M2). The flat breaststroke swimmers had the smallest stroke lengths for both males and females.

Table 2. Stroke frequency, stroke length, and average CM horizontal velocity

Swimmer	Stroke frequency (cycles/s)	Stroke length (m)	Av. CM velocity (m/s)
M1	0.59	2.04	1.20
M2	0.59	2.13	1.26
M3	0.70	1.72	1.20
F1	0.54	2.16	1.17
F2	0.65	1.55	1.01
F3	0.98	1.22	1.20

3.3 Pull, kick, glide, and deadspace times
The most important feature of the phase times was the very small duration of glide for swimmers F3 (0.07 s; 7% of the stroke cycle) and M3 (0.0 s). The other four subjects had glide phases between 0.46 s (30%) to 0.55 s (33%). This largely accounted for their small stroke frequencies and long stroke lengths compared to those of F3 and M3. Pull times expressed as a percentage of the stroke cycle were long for F3 (54.9%) and M3 (58.0%). The other four subjects had pull phases between 29.9% (F1) and 35.3% (M2). There were no obvious differences in deadspace or kick times that were related to the use of the wave action technique.

3.4 CM velocity
Maximum CM velocities ranged from 1.57 m/s (F1) to 1.77 m/s (F2). Minimum CM velocities ranged from 0.45 m/s (F1) to 0.86 m/s (M1). There was no clear trend with respect to the range of velocity and the use of the wave action technique. However, the most 'wavelike' swimmer (M1) had the greatest minimum (0.86 m/s) and smallest range (0.76 m/s). This was despite having a relatively long glide time (0.54 s). This indicated an efficient technique which minimised drag.

3.5 Trunk and thigh angles
There was considerable uniformity among the swimmers with respect to maximum trunk angles with the exception of F2 (28 degrees) who had a flat style of breaststroke and F1 (53 degrees) who had a very undulating style. The other squad members had maximum angles between 39 degrees (F3) and 46 degrees (M1). The maximum trunk angles occurred close (within 0.1 s) to the time of maximum shoulder elevation. Minimum trunk angles were generally close to zero and tended to occur during the glide phase immediately following the kick and lunge. For those with very short glide phases (F3 and M3) the minimum trunk angle was attained at the beginning of the pull phase.

Maximum thigh angles ranged from 54 degrees (F3) to 68 degrees (M2) and corresponded closely to the start of the kick. They also corresponded closely to the lowest velocity of the

CM indicating that retracting the legs was the major cause of loss of velocity during the breaststroke cycle. Swimmers tended to commence the recovery of their legs just before the maximum trunk angle was achieved. At the time of maximum trunk angle the thighs were still at a small angle to horizontal. This meant that the body had a natural curve.

Figure 1 shows that the wave action swimmer M1 attained a level and streamlined position following the lunge enabling a long glide without a great reduction in velocity. By contrast, the shanks and thighs of the flat swimmer F3 were not elevated enough to attain a level position. This swimmer was less streamlined and had a short glide phase.

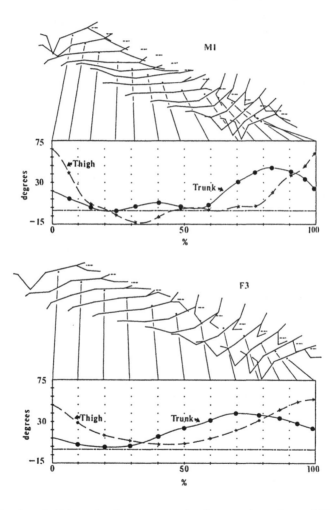

Fig. 1 Trunk and thigh angles for a wave action breaststroke swimmer M1 and a flat breaststroke swimmer F3.

4 References

1.   Muckenfuss, M. (1989) Catching the wave. *Swimming Technique*, August-October. 11-15.
2.   Persyn, U. (1991) Diagnosis of the movement and physical characteristics leading to feedback in the breaststroke, in *Competitive Swimming Barcelona and Beyond: Proceedings of the Pan Pacific International Swim Co Symposium* (ed. J.M. Hogg). Swim Alberta Association, Edmonton, August 26-28, 1991, pp. 30-62.
3.   Dempster, W.T. (1955) *Space Requirements of the Seated Operator.* (WADC TR 55-159), Wright-Patterson Air Force Base, OH.
4.   Troup, J.P. (1991) *International Center for Aquatics Research Annual: Studies by the International Center for Aquatic Research 1990-1991.* United States Swimming Press, Colorado Springs.

10 A METHOD TO ANALYZE KINEMATIC PARAMETERS DURING CRAWL SPRINT SWIMMING

W. WIRTZ*, K. WILKE*, J. KLAUCK** and B. LANGNICKEL
German Sports University, Cologne, Germany
*Institute of Aquatic Sports, **Institute of Biomechanics

Abstract
The purpose of this study was a) to evaluate the method of analyzing swimming motions during a race with two parallel moving cameras (PMC-method) and b) to gain an insight into the process of movement pattern changes during the 50 m crawl sprint. Ten swimmers were recorded and digitized from the left and right side by two parallel moving cameras during a 50 m crawl sprint. Wrist and hip were digitized in the beginning and at the end of the race and three-dimensional coordinates were calculated using the DLT method [1]. These results were compared to a 15 m crawl sprint with stationary cameras. Kinematic parameters of temporal and spatial pulling patterns of the arm (wrist) relative to the swimmers body were analyzed. Intraindividual differences were found in temporal parameters but not in the spatial patterns of the movements. The measurements from both the moving and stationary cameras showed nearly identical results; therefore, the PMC-method is useful for analyzing kinematic parameters in swimming within the events.
Keywords: Kinematic, Method, Sprint Swimming.

1 Introduction

Kinematic data of spatial and temporal development of pulling patterns during a race allows a better insight into different movement pattern changes. For this purpose, it is useful to have three-dimensional data of the swimmer during the whole race. In the 50 m crawl sprint speed decreases continously after a short period of maximal velocity. This decrease in speed is caused mainly by the reduction of the stroke frequency [2]. Parallel moving cameras (PMC-method) were able to analyze this more in detail.

2 Methods

The subjects involved in this study were 5 female and 5 male swimmers of regional and national level. The swimmers were 15 to 26 years of age and their maximal performance over 50 m freestyle ranged from 23.9 to 32.1 s. They started in a 50 m pool from the water-level. Two cameras, fixed on a platform, moved simultaneously parallel to the swimmer. Time measurement started by the push-off of the feet from the wall. Both video tapes were synchronized, digitized (25 Hz) and evaluated by special software programs (developed by the Institute of Biomechanics) using the DLT method. The three-dimensional wrist pulling pattern data were analyzed to define three linear measures: depth (y coordinate), width (z coordinate) and length (x coordinate). The absolute displacements of the swimmers in all planes were calculated between the displacement of the moving platform and the swimmers movement in relation to the platform. Velocity of the platform was determined by digitizing reference points fixed on a steel cable over 50 m. All kinematic parameters of the wrist relative to the swimmers body in the three planes were computed by the sum of the absolute horizontal (x) displacement of the hip and the absolute three-dimensional pathway of the wrist. The magnitude of the velocity was computed by the vectors of the three planes. The swimmer swam twice with 1 hour rest between the races and the results of the two trials were averaged. Additionally, two subjects swam one 15 m sprint recorded by stationary cameras. The differences of the two filming methods were evaluated by the absolute pulling patterns which were generated by the overlapping of the relative velocity of the pulling movement towards the body and the actual velocity of the swimmer. The motion of the arm relative to the body was independent from the swimmers velocity and used to describe kinematic differences in the event. The following parameters were analyzed in the beginning (b) and end (e) of the 50 m:

1. Data of a complete arm cycle (both arms): mean velocity of the swimmer (VCb, VCe), time (TCb, TCe) and stroke length (SLCb,SLCe).
2. Spatial kinematic parameters of one arm relative to the swimmers body:
   Stroke depth (SDb, SDe) and distance in the water (DWRb, DWRe).
3. Temporal kinematic parameters of one arm relative to the swimmers body:
   time in the water (TIWb, TIWe), time outside of the water (TOWb, TOWe), time of down- (TDRb,TDRe),back- and upward sweep (TBURb, TBURe), peak velocity in the water (PVRb, PVRe) and time to reach PVR (TPVRb, TPVRe).

The intraindividual results in the beginning and the end of the distance were statistically treated by using a paired t-test.

3 Results

3.1 Evaluation of the method
The two different methods of recording were assessed by the absolute pulling pattern of two swimmers who swam under both recording conditions (Figure 1).

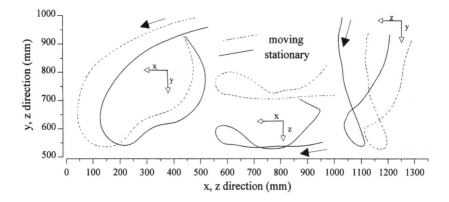

Figure 1. The absolute curve pattern (no. 9) of a left wrist
(view: side, bottom from underneath, frontal from ahead).

The results of the measured swimmers under both recording conditions showed nearly identical curve patterns.

3.2 Intraindividual differences

The average time of the two trials ranged between 25.5 and 34.0 s. All Swimmers showed a similar pulling pattern concerning the three-dimensional structure. The main pulling direction for all swimmers changed with the entry in the water from down-, to back- and upward (Figure 2). For the statistical treatment, the upward phase was added to the backward phase because its duration was too short for a single analysis.

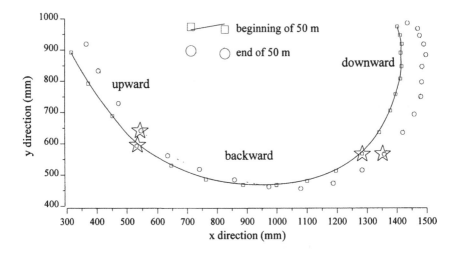

Figure 2. The sagittal plane of the right wrist during the race (no. 6).

The velocity of the wrist relative to the swimmers body (Figure 3) increased more or less till the end of the backward and beginning of the upward phase of the armstroke.

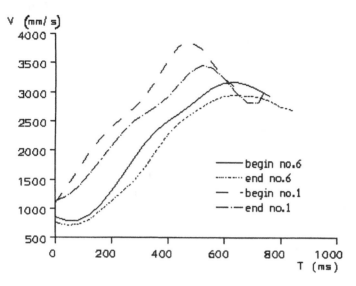

Figure 3. The relative velocity towards the body of the left wrist at the beginning and end of a 50 crawl sprint.

The statistical treatment of the individual results (Table 1) of the swimmers showed that the temporal factors (except TOW) changed and the spatial patterns remained nearly the same during the race (Table 2).

Table 1. Differences of kinematic parameters during a 50 m race

Subj.	VC	TC	SLC	TIW	TOW	TDR	TBUR	SD	DWR	PVR	TPVR
1 *	1.77	1.14	2.02	0.70	0.44	0.28	0.42	0.54	1.89	3.86	0.58
**	1.74	1.22	2.12	0.76	0.46	0.30	0.46	0.56	1.94	3.50	0.60
2	1.78	1.06	1.89	0.60	0.46	0.24	0.36	0.54	1.82	4.12	0.56
	1.73	1.08	1.87	0.62	0.46	0.24	0.38	0.56	1.82	4.02	0.58
3	1.76	1.06	1.86	0.68	0.38	0.32	0.36	0.51	1.68	3.79	0.62
	1.69	1.10	1.86	0.72	0.38	0.34	0.38	0.50	1.67	3.57	0.66
4	1.75	1.12	1.96	0.62	0.50	0.26	0.36	0.45	1.60	4.00	0.50
	1.69	1.14	1.92	0.68	0.46	0.28	0.40	0.41	1.65	3.64	0.50
5	1.63	1.30	2.12	0.72	0.58	0.36	0.36	0.39	1.44	3.44	0.64
	1.56	1.30	2.03	0.82	0.48	0.42	0.40	0.39	1.49	3.18	0.70
6	1.55	1.20	1.87	0.74	0.46	0.32	0.42	0.52	1.69	3.08	0.62
	1.51	1.28	1.93	0.82	0.46	0.36	0.46	0.50	1.76	2.94	0.66
7	1.55	1.04	1.61	0.64	0.40	0.26	0.38	0.44	1.56	3.28	0.54
	1.47	1.12	1.65	0.70	0.42	0.28	0.42	0.46	1.55	3.11	0.58
8	1.50	1.22	1.83	0.78	0.44	0.36	0.42	0.44	1.60	3.20	0.60
	1.48	1.32	1.95	0.84	0.48	0.38	0.46	0.44	1.64	3.17	0.65
9	1.45	1.38	2.00	0.78	0.60	0.32	0.46	0.42	1.57	3.06	0.70
	1.41	1.40	1.98	0.84	0.56	0.38	0.46	0.41	1.51	2.75	0.74
10	1.38	1.38	1.90	0.80	0.58	0.38	0.42	0.45	1.65	3.25	0.74
	1.36	1.52	2.06	0.88	0.64	0.42	0.46	0.43	1.60	3.10	0.78

* beginning, ** end

Table 2. Intraindividual differences of kinematic parameters in a 50 m race.

Kinematic Parameters	Beginning of the race		End of the race		Difference
	Mean	SD	Mean	SD	
VC	1.61	0.15	1.56	0.14	s
TC	1.19	0.13	1.25	0.14	s
SLC	1.90	0.14	1.94	0.13	ns
TIW	0.71	0.07	0.77	0.08	s
TOW	0.48	0.08	0.48	0.07	ns
TDR	0.31	0.05	0.34	0.06	s
TBUR	0.40	0.04	0.43	0.04	s
SD	0.46	0.06	0.47	0.05	ns
DWR	1.65	0.13	1.66	0.14	ns
PVR	3.51	0.40	3.30	0.38	s
TPVR	0.61	0.07	0.65	0.08	s

s = significant $p < 0.05$; ns = not significant $p > 0.05$

4 Discussion

The two methods of recording showed nearly identical curve patterns. The PMC-method appears to be a useful tool to analyze kinematic data. The spatial curve patterns relative to the swimmers body remained equal during a 50 m race and the temporal curve patterns changed significantly. This (Table 2, Figure 3) seemed to be responsible for the loss in swimming speed within the race and. could be reasoned by the energy supply (ATP production/time) which decreases very quickly in sprinting events [3]. The interindividual decrease in swimming speed during the race didn't vary much because the swimmers decelerate their speed in similar temporal dimensions (Table 1 and 2). This confirmed the results of an investigation of Zimmerman [2] with highly skilled swimmers (n = 117). Therefore the ability to swim very fast over an extremly short distance seems to be the basic factor for sprint swimming. The ability to mantain this speed seems to be less important. This depends either on biological abilities to produce energy or the speed endurance training was not effective enough to reduce the loss of speed during the race. In future this could be perhaps influenced by developing special speed endurance training methods and devices especially for 50 m sprinter.

4 References

1. Abdel-Aziz, Y.I. and Karar, H.M. (1971) Direct linear transformation: from comparator coordinates into object coordinates in close-range photogrammetry. *Proceedings ASPUI Symposium on Close Range Photogrammetry*, Church Falls, pp.1-19.
2. Zimmermann, F. (1990) *Zyklusweg- und Frequenzmessung auf der 50 m-Sprintstrecke im Kraulschwimmen.* Diplomarbeit, Deutsche Sporthochschule Köln.
3. Heck, H. (1990) *Energiestoffwechsel und medizinische Leistungsdiagnostik.* Studienbrief 8 der Trainerakademie Köln, Schorndorf.

11 BIOMECHANICAL HIGHLIGHTS OF WORLD CHAMPION AND OLYMPIC SWIMMERS

J.M. CAPPAERT, D.L. PEASE and J.P. TROUP
U.S. Swimming, International Center for Aquatic Research
University of Colorado, Colorado Springs, USA.

1 Overview

During the 1991 World Championships and the 1992 Ólympic Games, swimmers in lane four were videotaped with a four camera system (two above water and two cameras underwater) at approximately the 40-45m mark of the pool. The four videotapes were digitized to create a 14 segment, three-dimensional model of the body during one stroke cycle [1]. The center of mass (using cadaver data [2]) and several body position angles were calculated. Hand reaction forces were calculated [3]. Landmark data were differentiated and all parameters were used to described stroke technique. The comparisons below are made within a gender and within a race distance.

Keywords: Three-dimensional analysis, elite swimmer comparisons.

2 Elite vs. Non-elite Swimmer Comparisons

2.1 Butterfly

Trunk angle, as defined by the mid-shoulder, mid-hip and the forward horizontal, seemed to be as important variable in butterfly swimming. Elite butterfliers tended to have lower trunk angles when compared to non-elite. The lower trunk angle position was related to both elbow extension and the percent of propulsive force in the finish phase of the stroke. Butterfly swimmers who had a lower trunk angle were able to extend the elbows more during the finish phase of the pulling pattern which allowed them to direct a higher percentage of those forces in the propulsive direction. Another benefit of a lower trunk angle could be that the body was more streamlined at that point in the stroke.

For an individual example, during the Olympic Games 100m butterflier Xiaohong Wang and a swimmer from the preliminary heats showed a difference in maximum trunk angle (Figure 1; Wang = 32.8 deg, non-elite swimmer = 50.1 deg). The pulling patterns were different between the two swimmers as well. Wang was more symmetrical between arms than the heats swimmer (propelling efficiencies = Wang: 35.3% right arm, 32.2% left arm; non-elite swimmer: 40.2% right arm, 30.1% left arm). The non-elite swimmer emphasized the insweep phase for propulsion whereas Wang had propulsive finish phases for both arms. Wang maximized the propulsiveness of the finish phases for each arm by extending the elbows and wrists.

The strengths of elite butterfliers stroke are: 1) low trunk angle, 2) symmetrical pulling patterns, and 3) extended elbows and wrists during the finish phase of the pulling pattern.

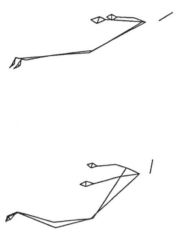

Figure 1. Trunk angle differences in butterfly. Wang (top) vs. Heats Swimmer (bottom).

2.2 Backstroke

Body roll from the shoulders and hips was a significant in the backstroke. Olympic gold medal winner, Krisztina Egerszegi, had symmetrical body roll (Figure 2). This was quantified in the amount of shoulder and hip roll (max shoulder and hip roll angles were 48.8 deg and 45 deg, respectively), and the timing of her rotation (shoulders and hips reached their maximum angles at approximately the same time). Non-elite swimmers from the preliminary heats tended to have opposite rotation from the shoulders and hips. For example, a non-elite swimmer had a maximum shoulder roll angle of 45.6 degrees while her hips were rolling downward at -39.7 deg (see Figure 2). This opposite body roll has two potential disadvantages: 1) it is not as streamlined, and 2) this body position tends to decrease the use of the trunk muscles during the pulling pattern.

Elite backstrokers had large knee range of motion (61 deg) which in turn gave the foot a large range of motion to produce propulsive forces during the kick. Non-elite swimmers do not seem to emphasize the kick as heavily as seen in a non-elite swimmer who flexed her knees through a range of motion of 43.6 degrees.

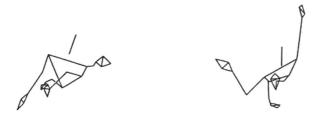

Figure 2. Body roll differences in backstroke, Egerszegi (right) vs. Heats swimmer (left).

The strengths of elite backstrokers are: 1) symmetrical body roll, and 2) emphasizing the kick by flexing the knee through a range of motion of over 70 degrees.

2.3 Breaststroke
A key factor in the breaststroke is timing. There was a difference in the timing of the kick between the 200m world record holder, Michael Barrowman, and most of the swimmers in the preliminary heats. Specifically, Barrowman recovered his legs quickly and was ready to kick as his head entered the water. In comparison, a non-elite swimmer fully recovered his arms, and his body was almost horizontal before he began his kick. This timing difference had a dramatic affect on the forward swimming velocity of the two swimmers. Barrowman's quick leg recovery and kick minimized the time spent in the deadspace of the arm and leg recoveries. Barrowman's hip velocity decreased for only approximately 0.25 seconds and his center of mass velocity was fairly well maintained (Figure 3). In contrast, the slowness of the leg recovery for the non-elite swimmer caused not only the hip velocity but also the center of mass velocity to decrease for approximately 0.5 seconds.

Additionally, Barrowman had a very effective pulling pattern as evidenced by his propelling efficiency (38.5% right arm , 35.2% left arm). Despite a faster turnover rate Barrowman had approximately the same amount of propulsive time as the non-elite swimmer.

The strengths of elite breaststrokers are: 1) whole body streamlining throughout all phases of the stroke cycle, 2) the timing of the arm and leg recoveries, and 3) high propelling efficiency of the pulling patterns.

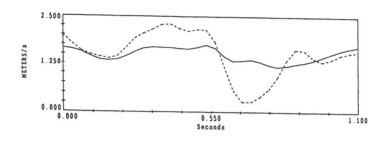

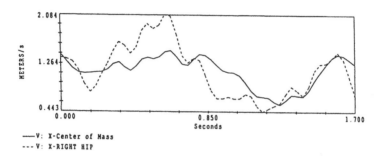

—V: X-Center of Mass
--- V: X-RIGHT HIP

Figure 3. Center of mass and hip velocity differences in breaststroke, Barrowman (top) vs. Heats swimmer (bottom).

2.4 Freestyle

There are a few key body position variables that distinguish elite from non-elite freestylers. As in backstroke, elite freestylers had symmetrical body roll in that both the shoulders and hips are rolling in the same direction (for example, Alexandre Popov shoulder roll = 43.1 deg, hip roll = 40.9 deg). Non-elite freestylers tended to have adequate shoulder roll, but opposite hip roll (a non-elite swimmer shoulder roll = 43.3 deg, hip roll = -33.2 deg).

Figure 4 highlights differences in pulling pattern, specifically the elbow position. Elite swimmers were able to keep their elbows high during the catch and the beginning of the insweep phase, whereas non-elite swimmer lead with their elbow during those phases. Pulling pattern force analyses revealed that elite freestylers used less propulsive forces and higher propelling efficiencies than non-elite to swim faster velocities. Additionally, elite swimmers had better whole body streamlining.   Therefore, non-elite swimmers may have needed more propulsive force to compensate for poor body position.

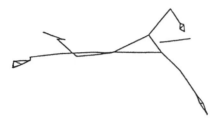

Figure 4. Correct elbow position in freestyle.

The strengths of elite freestylers are: 1) symmetrical body roll, 2) high elbow position during the catch, the beginning of the insweep, and 3) efficient force application.

3 Summary

In summary, elite athletes do not only possess great strength and power which accelerates them through the water. These athletes have the ability to apply that power to the water effectively through proper technique (higher propelling efficiency). There also seems to be the trend that elite athletes do not use significant higher propulsive forces from their arms and legs. Rather, they have better whole body streamlining which reduces the drag forces from the water. Therefore, they can achieve faster swimming velocities using similar overall propulsion as non-elite athletes.

4 References

1.   Cappaert, J.M., D.L. Pease and J.P. Troup (1991). Methodology for over water recovery and underwater stroke pattern analysis in swimming, in *Proceedings of the Second International Olympic Committee World Congress on Sport Sciences,* Barcelona, Spain.
2.   Dempster, W.T. (1955). Space requirements of the seated operator, in *WADC Technical Report,* Wright-Patterson Air Force Base, Ohio.
3.   Schleihauf, R.E. (1979). A hydrodynamic analysis of swimming propulsion, in, *Swimming III: Proceedings of the Third International Symposium of Biomechanics in Swimming,* (eds. J. Terauds & W. Bedingfield), University Park Press, Baltimore, pp. 70-109.

PART THREE

MEDICAL ASPECTS

12 SWIMMERS' SHOULDER: EMG OF THE ROTATORS DURING A FLUME TEST

K.M. MONTEIL*, A.H. ROUARD*, A.B. DUFOUR**, J.M. CAPPAERT*** and J.P. TROUP***

*Laboratoire de la Performance, C.R.I.S., Lyon France
**Laboratoire d'analyse de données et de biométrie, C.R.I.S., Lyon France
***U.S. Swimming, University of Colorado, Colorado Springs, USA.

Abstract
The aim of this investigation was to study the relationships between the rotators cuff of the shoulder during an exercise bout conducted in front crawl in a flume. Nine male swimmers realised a 400 yards front crawl at their maximal intensity. Electrical activities of six rotators of the shoulder were recorded using dual fine wire electrodes during the first and last five seconds of the test. The electrical signal was integrated, averaged at 50 Hz and normalized in relation to the maximal dynamic contraction obtained during the swim for each subject. Data analysis used standardized principal component analyses. Results showed a great discrepancy between the subjects, underlining the individual electrical responses of the studied population. No predominance of a muscular group (external or internal rotators) was observed. The relationships between the muscles were different at the beginning and at the end of the test. As a result, the activity of an external (or internal) rotator could not be assumed as representative of the activity of other external (or internal) rotators. Muscles could be activated all through the phases with different functions, which could not be identified using the EMG methods.
Keywords: EMG, exhaustion, shoulder, swimming.

1 Introduction

In swimming, since Ikai et al. [1], superficial muscles have been widely investigated using surface electrode. As noticed by Vaday and Nemessuri [2], "the main role of the propulsive power of free-style swimming is played by muscles of the shoulder girdle". Other studies confirmed that the shoulder joint was the more linked to the propulsion [3] and that joint was strained by various mechanisms as a high repetition rate [4]. Moreover the muscles of the shoulder provided alternately "the propelling force and repositionned the arm for the next thrust" [4]. This joint is mobilized all through the front crawl stroke. As a result, the number of the swimmers complaining about pain after years of training [5] increased. This pain has been named the shoulder impigement syndrome "SIS", and defined as a "chronic irritation of the humeral head and rotator cuff on the coracoacromial arch during the abduction of the shoulder" [6]. Since the last decade, this joint was more analised, but most of the muscles of the girdle shoulder belong to the deep part of the body and required fine-wire electrodes.

Only few studies were conducted using this invasive method [7], [8], since the first one realised in swimming [9].

From these previous studies, and in regard to the description of the shoulder mechanics in front crawl [6], the external and the internal rotators seemed to be activated all through the stroke. Then the muscular activity through the aquatic stroke phases and the relationships between the rotators cuff during a front crawl test conducted to exhaustion in a flume will be analysed.

2 Methods

2.1 Population
Nine male volunteer swimmers were involved in this study. Their anthropometrical characteristics were reported in table 1.

Table 1. Anthropometrical characteristics of the population

	Age (years)	Height (cm)	Weight (kg)	Body fat (%)
Mean	23.8	184.0	77.9	9.4
1 Standard dev.	4.5	5.0	5.8	1.1
Range	17-30	175-193	70.3-90.7	7.8-10.8

For height and weight parameters, population appeared to be homogeneous, whereas for age and body fat values were rather extended.

2.2 Test and data acquisition
The test took place in a flume (swimming treadmill), where the subject stayed on the same place while the water was moving. Each swimmer realised the test in front crawl at his maximal intensity corresponding to a 400 yards. The test was over when the swimmer could not keep the pace and was flowing back in the flume.

During the test, the electrical activities of six shoulder's rotators were recorded with dual fine-wire electrodes. The studied muscles were external rotators (m. supraspinatus, m. infraspinatus and m. terres minor) and internal rotators (m. subscapularis, m. pectoralis major pars clavicular and m. latissimus dorsi). Muscles were inserted according to Delagi et al. orders [10]. The system used for recording the muscular activities took into account ISEK report [11]. Silmutaneously, two underwater video cameras (30 Hz) filmed the subject, in order to determine the aquatic phases of the stroke.

Data were collected during the first five seconds (initial condition) and last ones (final condition) of the swimming test. One arm stroke was studied for each condition.

2.3 Data treatment
Electrical signals were rectified, integrated, averaged on 50 Hz sequences and normalized to the maximal dynamic contraction recorded during the test for each swimmer.

The aquatic phases of the stroke were divided into three phases [12]. These phases were divided from the motion of the fingertips in the frontal plan into catch (from the hand entry into the water to the more external point of the hand), insweep (from the more external point to the more internal point of the hand) and finish (from the more internal point to the hand exit).

2.4 Statistical methods
A standardized principal component analysis (PCA) based on the correlation matrix of the EMG data was computed, in order to determine relations between the rotators muscles and to find a simple view of the complex EMG phenomena [13].

3 Results

A standardized PCA was computed for each condition of the test.

3.1 Initial condition
The first two components accounted for 65.84 % of the variation for PCA (Fig. 1), and pointed out the good representation of the studied variables.

m1: m. pectoralis major
     pars clavicular
m2: m. supraspinatus
m3: m. infraspinatus
m4: m. teres minor
m5: m. latissimus dorsi
m6: m. subscapularis

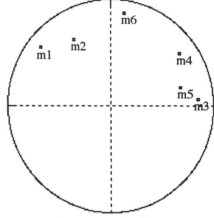

Fig. 1. Correlations between muscular activities and the two first principal components.

The first axis (horizontal axis) was mainly defined by antagonists muscles, m. infraspinatus (m3), m. teres minor (m4) and m. latissimus dorsi (m5). This result indicated that these muscles were activated similarly. An opposition of activity can be observed between these muscles and the m. pectoralis major pars clavicular (m1). The second axis (vertical axis) was composed by the m. subscapularis (m6). This muscle seemed to be indepedent of the other muscles.

From the axes 1 and 2 (Fig. 2) the muscular activity of the subjects can be observed. The representation pointed out that subjects activated preferential muscles. For example, the swimmer s2, in regard to his location, presented an important activity of the muscular group composed by the m. infraspinatus, the m. teres minor and the m. latissimus dorsi. The swimmer s6 favorised the activation of the m. pectoralis major pars clavicular. The swimmer s5 did not seem to activate the m. subscapularis. Various individual muscular responses can be noticed. Looking at the muscular activity through the aquatic phases of the stroke, three different groups of swimmers emerged. Some swimmers had few variations of the muscular activities of their shoulder rotators (subjects s1, s3, s4 and s8), presenting small trajectories (point phases closed to each other). Other swimmers (s2, s5, s7 and s9) presented variations in their muscular activity through the aquatic phases. These swimmers presented trajectories rather extended, their phases point being spaced out.

For example, the swimmer s2 showed an increase of the m. subscapularis activity during the insweep phase, as the swimmer s9. The swimmer s7 recorded an important activity of the m. subscapularis during the catch and the insweep phases with an increase of the activity of the m. infraspinatus, m. teres minor and m. latissimus dorsi during the insweep one. Finally the swimmer s6 tended to have a decreasing muscular activity all through the phase.

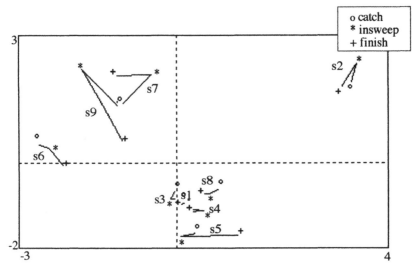

Fig. 2. Subjects representation on the first factorial plan.

3.2 Final condition

The first two components presented a good representation of the variables, with a 64.50 % value of the variation for PCA (Fig. 3).

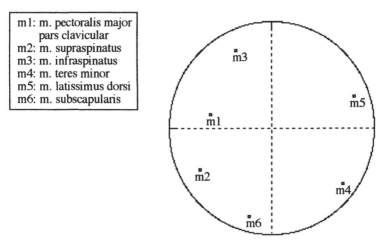

Fig. 3.   Correlations between muscular activities and the two first principal components.

Contrarly to the initial condition, no predominance of a muscular groups seemed to be pointed out. The first axis (horizontal axis) was determined by the muscular activity of the m. teres minor (m4) and the m. latissimus dorsi (m5). The activity of these two muscles seemed to be opposed to the activity of the m. pectoralis major pars clavicular (m1) and m. supraspinatus (m2). The second axis (vertical axis) was defined by the M infraspinatus (m3) and the m. subscapularis (m6). The muscular activities of these muscles were opposed and independent of the other muscles.

From the axes 1 and 2 (Fig. 4) the muscular activity of the subjects all through the phases can be studied.

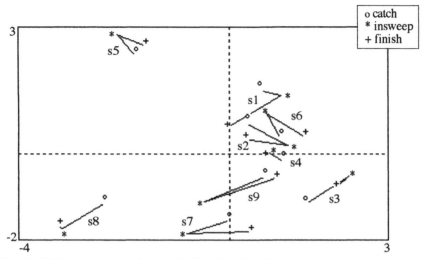

Fig. 4. Subjects representation on the first factorial plan.

Four groups of subjects emerged concerning the muscles activated. The swimmer s5 had an important activity of the m. infraspinatus. The swimmers s8 and s7 recorded an important activity of the m. subscapularis. The swimmer s3 presented an important activity of the m. teres minor. Other subjects did not seem to activate a specific muscle. Moreover, all the subjects showed a specific activity all through the aquatic stroke phases (all the trajectories were rather extended). For the population, the insweep phase seemed to be the one who pointed out a different activity compared to the catch or the finish parts of the stroke.

4 Discussion

The subjects presented various muscular activities during the initial and the final conditions. They did not mainly activate the same muscles and presented variations through the aquatic phases of the stroke. This result underlined the individual electrical responses of the swimmers, which confirmed previous studies [14]. Each standardized principal component analysis pointed out various muscular groups. These muscular relationships differed in the initial and in the final test conditions where no predominance of a muscular group was observed. From the anatomical assumptions, we were expected to find a similar activity between muscles with a same function. For example, we supposed that the activity of an internal rotator would be representative of the activity of the other internal rotators of the shoulder. This was not the case. This result could be explained by the fact that some of the studied muscles could be activated in a different functional role according to their anatomical location [15]. For example, the m. latissimus dorsi could be activated as an internal rotator, but also as an adductor or an extensor of the shoulder. An important muscular activity all through the aquatic phases of the stroke was noticed. This result infirmed previous findings [7], [8]. These authors observed that muscles did not fire all through the stroke but during some phases. The rather important activation obtained, could be due that some of the studied muscles could be recruited as propulsor and/or as stabilizer of the shoulder as described in previous study [16]. Clarys and Cabri [17] noticed that "a wide range of statements have been made from elementary anatomical knowledge and functional reasoning". Front crawl stroke is a complex motion, and anatomical and functional approaches appeared not to be sufficient to analyse muscular activity. The EMG did not lead to the distinction of the part of activity due to the various functional role of a muscle.

5 Conclusion

Results underlined the individual muscular activities of the subjects. Moreover, no predominance of a muscular group (external or internal rotators) was found, and the relationships between the muscles were different during the initial and the final conditions of the test. Then the activity of an external (or an internal) rotator could not be assumed as representative of the activity of other external (or internal rotators). Muscles could be activated all through the phases with different functions, which could not be identified using EMG methods.

6 References

1. Ikai, M., Ishii, K. and Miyashita, M. (1964) An electromyography study of swimming. *Research Journal of Physical Education*, 7, pp. 47-54.
2. Vaday, M. and Nemessuri, M. (1971) Motor pattern of freestyle swimming. *Biomechanics of Swimming*, (ed. L. Lewillie and J.P. Clarys), Brussels: Université Libre de Bruxelles, pp. 167-173.
3. Welch, J.H. (1974) A kinematic analysis of world-class stroke swimmers. *Biomechanics IV*, (ed. R.C. Nelson and C.A. Morehouse), Baltimore: University Park Press, pp. 217-222.
4. Perry, J. (1983) Anatomy and biomechanics of the shoulder in throwing, swimming, gymnastics and tennis. *Clinics in Sports Medicine*, 2, pp. 247-270.
5. Beekman, K.M. and Hay, J.G. (1988) Characteristics of the front crawl techniques of swimmers with shoulder impigement syndrome. *Journal of Swimming Research*, 4, pp. 11-14.
6. Richardson, A.B., Jobe, F.W. and Collins, H.R. (1980) The shoulder in competitive swimming. *American Journal of Sports Medicine*, 8, pp. 159-163.
7. Moynes, D.R., Perry, J., Antonelli, D.J. and Jobe, F.W. (1986) Electromyography and motion analysis of the upper extremity in sports. *Physical Therapy*, 66, pp. 1905-1911.
8. Nuber, G.W., Jobe, F.W., Perry, J., Moynes, D.R. and Antonelli, D.J. (1986) Fine wire electromyography analysis of muscles of the shoulder during swimming. *American Journal of Sports Medicine*, 14, pp. 7-11.
9. Okamoto, T. and Wolf, S.L. (1979) Underwaterrecording of muscular activity using fine-wire electrodes. *Swimming III*, (ed. J. Terauds and E.W. Bedingfield), Baltimore: University Park Press, pp. 160-166.
10. Delagi, E.F., Perotto, A., Iazzetti, J. and Morrison, D. (1980) *Anatomic guide for the electromyographer*, CC Thomas Publisher Springfield, Illinois, U.S.A.
11. Winter, D.A., Rau, G., Kadefors, R., Broman, H. and De Luca, C.J. (1980) *Units terms and standards in the reporting of EMG research,* Report of the ISEK.
12. Maglischo, C.W., Maglischo, E.W., Sharp, R.L., Zier, D.J. and Katz, A. (1984) Tethered and non tethered crawl swimming. *Sports Biomechanics*, (ed. J. Terauds, K. Barthels, E. Kreighbaum, R. Mannand J. Crakes), Del Mar: Research center for sports, pp. 163-176.

13. Kendall, M. (1975) *Multivariate analysis.* Ed. Griffin, London. Chap. 2.
14. Piette, G. and Clarys, J.P. (1979) Telemetric electromyography of the front crawl movement. *Swimming III*, (ed. J. Terauds and E.W. Bedingfield), Baltimore/University Park Press, pp. 153-159.
15. Brizon, J. and Castaing, J. (1953) Muscles du membre supérieur. *Les feuillets d'anatomie*, fascicule IV, (ed. Maloine S.A.), Paris, pp. 1-123.
16. Kreighbaum, E. and Barthels, K.M. (1990) *Biomechanics: a qualitative approach for studying human movement.* Ed. Macmillan Publishing Company, New York, 3rd edition: Chap. 4.
17. Clarys, J.P. and Cabri, J. (1993) Electromyography and the study of sports movements: A review. *Journal of Sports Sciences*, 11, pp. 379-448.

13 COMPARISON OF SHOULDER INJURY IN COLLEGIATE AND MASTERS LEVEL SWIMMERS

D. STOCKER, M. PINK and F.W. JOBE
Biomechanics Laboratory, Centinela Hospital
Inglewood, California, USA

Abstract

All ages and levels are represented in the one-hundred million Americans who classify themselves as a swimmer. To investigate the differences between young, highly competitive collegiate swimmers and older, less elite swimmers a survey questionnaire was distributed to 100 collegiate and 100 master's swim teams. Several questions and possible predisposing factors associated with "swimmers shoulder" were investigated. Results revealed that the collegiate group swam the higher yardage as well as faster times in two distances of freestyle swimming. However, the collegiate and master's group reported similar percentages of those experiencing shoulder pain lasting three or more weeks, despite the lesser distances and intensities associated with the later group. Chi-square analysis revealed no association between shoulder pain and perceived level of flexibility, hand paddle usage or breathing side for either group. Over 50% of the swimmers with shoulder pain in both groups, perceived that increased intensities and/or distance provoked shoulder pain, indication that fatigue may be the issue to focus upon. Strengthening the muscles of the shoulder provides a strong defense against injury, as fatigue of the shoulder muscles may be the initial antecedent to "swimmers shoulder." These results give the swimmer, coach and medical practitioner feedback to consider when encountered with a swimmer of any age or level.

Keywords: Collegiate, injury, masters, shoulder, swimmer

1 Introduction

"Swimmers shoulder," typically used to describe any type of shoulder discomfort in the swimmer, is also the sports most common orthopedic complaint.

Since all ages and levels are represented in the one hundred million Americans who classify themselves as a swimmer [1], the need to investigate the incidence of shoulder pain in swimmers other than the young and very elite is evident. Three unavoidable factors influencing swimmers shoulder for any age or level swimmer are: 1) swimming demands an extremely high repetition rate of shoulder revolution, 2) swimming will take the shoulder to extremes of range of motion (ROM), 3) swimming requires the generation of high muscular forces on the shoulder in order to sustain the forward propulsive effort.

Several factors related to swimmers shoulder and associated training regimes have been implicated in the literature on shoulder injury [2,3,4,5,6,7].

The purpose of this survey study was to compare the swimming profiles of young, elite, collegiate swimmers versus older, less elite masters swimmers, as well as, to assess the correlation between previously described risk factors and "swimmers shoulder."

Comparison of the two populations provides insight and feedback for the coach and clinical practitioner to consider when a swimmer, of any age or level, presents with the common complaint of shoulder pain.

2 Methods

This study utilized a two page questionnaire which was sent to 100 randomly selected collegiate and masters swim teams. All collegiate swimmers competed under National Collegiate Athletic Association (NCAA), division I, II, or III guidelines. The beginning portion of the survey hosted the demographic data and continued with questions regarding their swimming routines and estimated weekly yardage.

Performance profiles were determined by asking questions regarding their current race time for 50 and 1,000 yards, and estimates of weekly yardage. An additional question asked whether they considered their body joints to be flexible, tight or average.

Page two of the survey delineated those with painful shoulders and made further inquiry into actions preceding and in response to the discomfort.

3 Results

Five hundred thirty-two collegiate swimmers and 395 masters swimmers returned the survey, making the response rate slightly over eighteen percent. Descriptive data for both groups are shown below.

Table 1. Descriptive Data on Collegiate & Masters Swimmers

	Collegiate	Masters
Average age (yrs)	19.5	41.5
Average age of entry into swimming (yrs)	9.1	22.1
Average age of entry into swimming (yrs) for swimmers with shoulder pain	8.8	25.1
Total years of consistent swimming	10.1	12.1
Swim sessions per week	8.6	4.0
Estimated wks/yr 6000 + yards	40.6	42.0

Distribution of estimated weekly yardage in 1,000 yard categories revealed that the largest percentage (26%) of collegiate swimmers swam between 40 and 50 thousand yards per week and the largest percentage (48%) of the masters population swam between 10 and 20 thousand yards per week.

Forty-six percent of the collegiate group reported incorporating paddles in their workouts while 28% of the masters group incorporated paddles.

Performance time breakdown for 50 and 1000 yards of freestyle swimming is shown below.

Table 2. Performance times for 50 and 1000 yards of freestyle swimming

50 Yards			1000 Yards		
	College	Masters		College	Masters
< 20 seconds	1%	0%	< 9 minutes	23%	0%
20-22 seconds	28%	2%	9-11 minutes	47%	22%
23-24 seconds	30%	10%	12-13 minutes	26%	31%
25-25 seconds	25%	18%	14-15 minutes	3%	19%
27-28 seconds	11%	14%	16-17 minutes	0%	15%
29-30 seconds	4%	16%	18-19 minutes	1%	7%
31-40 seconds	1%	33%	20> minutes	0%	6%
40> seconds	0%	7%			

Response from joint flexibility inquiry indicated similar distribution patterns of tight, average, and flexible subjective joint flexibility across both groups.

Both groups reported that nearly 50% of the swimmers sustained a swimming related shoulder injury. Forty-seven percent of the college and 48% of the masters swimmers claimed to have experienced shoulder pain lasting three weeks or more and in turn forced them to cease or alter their swimming routines.

When swimmers with shoulder pain were delineated from the entire group the percentages of subjective joint flexibility varied only slightly from those reported on swimmers without shoulder pain.

Fifty-five percent of the college swimmers with shoulder pain opted to seek medical intervention versus 39% of the masters swimmers.

Chi-square analysis revealed no statistically significant probability of breathing side or hand paddle usage having an association with shoulder pain (p>.05).

Another chi-square analysis, executed on those with shoulder pain revealed no statistically significant probability of an association between shoulder pain and subjective level of joint flexibility (p>.05).

An increase in intensity and or distance was self perceived to provoke the shoulder pain in over 50% of both college and masters swimmers.

4 Discussion

The mean age of the masters swimmer (41.5 years), compared to the college swimmer (19.5 years), is indicative of the long-term participatory rate of swimming while the similar percentage of collegiate and masters swimmers (47 and 48%, respectively) who experienced shoulder pain lasting three or more weeks indicates that "swimmers shoulder" is not a condition unique to the more elite or collegiate level swimmer. This reinforces the importance of attention to shoulder injuries sustained in the older population along with the need for further insight into their training routines.

Despite the faster swim times and more than double weekly yardage reported by the collegiate group both groups reported a similar amount of weeks out of the year in which they swam 6,000 yards or more, indicating that while the masters group may not train as intensely as the collegiate group they do train with equal consistency.

We found no probability of association between breathing side and side of shoulder pain in both groups. The similar flexibility percentages reported in college and masters swimmers with shoulder pain suggests that advancing years are not necessarily concomitant with perceived excessive joint tightness in swimmers. Furthermore, this suggests that level of flexibility may not be a determinant of susceptibility to injury.

Conversely, another study utilizing elite swimmers revealed that those incorporating stretching into their routines aggravated existing shoulder pain [6]. Forcing the shoulder into positions of extreme range of motion (ROM) can potentially damage the joint structure [8,9,10,11]. For a swimmer, maintaining adequate flexibility is necessary since it permits maximal stroke efficiency and coordination [10], however, caution should be implemented so as not to overstretch, especially in the anterior capsule of the shoulder. The effectiveness of proper warm up prior to swimming, for any age of level swimmer should not be ignored; however, coaches and swimmers should steer clear of the notion that greater flexibility will guarantee injury-free swimming and adhere to the idea that mobility must strike a balance with stability.

Since over 50% of the swimmers with shoulder pain in both groups perceived provocation with increased intensities and/or distance, fatigue may be the condition to avoid and focus upon. Recent electromyographic (EMG) data reveals that during freestyle swimming two muscles of the shoulder, the subscapularis and serratus anterior, are active throughout the stroke cycle and therefore, susceptible to fatigue [12]. Fatigue of these muscles potentially could cause the swimmer to alter his/her stroke, thereby interrupting smooth scapulohumeral rhythm. This asynchronous rhythm may trigger the shoulder continuum of overuse, progressing to microtrauma, instability and impingement [13].

In addition, quite commonly in strength programs used by swimmers, the muscles which provide propulsion, the pectoralis major and latissimus dorsi, are the focus and the muscles which provide shoulder girdle stability, the rotator cuff and scapular rotator muscles, are generally ignored. Ironically, it is the muscles that provide stability that are most prone to fatigue, namely the subscapularis and serratus anterior [12]. Special attention to these two critical muscles in a strengthening program would be advantageous to any swimmer. Coaches and swimmers should also closely monitor swim sessions and make sure to rest or change strokes when fatigue brought on by intense or overdistance swimming may bring about deterioration of the correct swimming mechanics or a sloppy stroke [4,5,8,14].

Hand paddles have been linked to shoulder pain in several studies [3,4,7]. In this study no statistically significant probability of association emerged when analyzing hand paddle usage and shoulder pain; however, the additional strain on the shoulder imposed by hand paddles may further fatigue an already susceptible shoulder. Therefore, one would be wise to limit the use of paddles as well as avoid using paddles late in a swim session when the muscles are most prone to fatigue.

The higher percentage of collegiate swimmers who opted to seek medical intervention may be due to the generally higher stakes involved. A collegiate swimmer may have scholarships and team pressures encouraging a rapid recovery.

These results give the coach and medical practitioner feedback on factors to consider when encountered with a swimmer, of any age or level, with the common complaint of "swimmers shoulder."

5 Summary

Response from a two page questionnaire sent to 100 collegiate and 100 master swim teams provided insight into training routines, shoulder injury rates and possible predisposing factors. Information collected on each groups performance time revealed the collegiate group to be swimming much higher weekly yardage and more than double the amount of workouts per week.

The similar percentage of collegiate and masters swimmers (47 and 48%, respectively) who experienced shoulder pain lasting three weeks or more, however, indicates that "swimmers shoulder" is not a condition unique only to the young, more competitive swimmer despite the lesser intensities and distances associated with the later group.

No association was found between shoulder pain and perceived level of flexibility, hand paddle usage or breathing side for either group.

Over 50% of those with shoulder pain in both groups reported provocation following an increase in swimming intensity and/or distance. This information, backed with current EMG data supports the notion that fatigue may be the major issue.

Implementing a strengthening program, with particular emphasis on the subscapularis and serratus anterior, the muscles most prone to fatigue, may be the swimmers best defense against shoulder injury.

6 References

1. Maglischo, E.W. (1993) Swimming Even Faster, Mayfield Publishing Co., Mountain View California.
2. Greipp, J.F. (1985) Swimmers' shoulder: The influence of flexibility and weight training. Physician and Sportsmedicine, Vol. 13, No. 8. pp. 92-105.
3. Hall, G. (1980) Hand paddles may cause shoulder pain. Swimming World, Vol. 21, No. 10. pp. 9-11.
4. Johnson, D. (1988) In swimming, shoulder the burden. Sportcare and Fitness, pp. 24-30.
5. Johnson, J.E., Sim, F.H. and Scott, S.G. (1987) Musculoskeletal injuries in competitive swimmers. Mayo Clinic Proceedings, No. 62. pp. 289-304.
6. McMaster, W.C. and Troup, J. (1993) A survey of interfering shoulder pain in United States competitive swimmers. American Journal of Sports Medicine, Vol. 21, No. 1. pp. 67-70.
7. Richardson, A.B., Jobe, F.W. and Collins, H.R. (1980) The shoulder in competitive swimming. American Journal of Sports Medicine, No. 8. pp. 159-163
8. Cuillo, J.V. and Stevens, G.G. (1989) The prevention and treatment of injuries to the shoulder in swimming. Sports Medicine, No. 7. pp. 182-204.
9. Kuland, D.N. and Tottossy, M. (1983) Warm up, strength and power. Orthopaedic Clinic of North America, Vol. 14, No. 2. pp. 427-448.
10. Marino, M. (1984) Profiling Swimmers. Clinic in Sports Medicine, Vol. 3, No. 1. pp. 211-229.
11. Shellock, F.G. and Prentice, W.E. (1985) Warming-up and stretching for improved physical performance and prevention of sports related injuries. Sports Medicine No. 2. pp. 267-278.
12. Scovazzo, M.L., Browne, A., Pink, M., Jobe, F.W. and Kerrigan, J. (1991) The painful shoulder during freestyle swimming: An electromyographic cinematographic analysis of twelve muscles. American Journal of Sports Medicine Vol. 19, No. 6. pp. 557-582.
13. Pink, M. and Jobe, F.W. (1991) Shoulder injuries in athletes. Orthopaedics, Vol. 11, No. 6. pp. 39-47.
14. Safran, M.R., Seaber, A.V. and Garrett, W.E. (1989) Warm-up and muscular injury prevention. An update Sports Medicine, Vol. 8, No. 4, pp. 239-249.

14 MEDICAL AIDS TO IMPROVE TRAINING

W.C. MCMASTER
University of California - Irvine
Department of Orthopaedic Surgery, Orange, California

Abstract
That swimming is not a high injury sport is corroborated by epidemiologic studies. [1] Injury can impede the ability of the athlete to progress in training and thereby attain a positive training effect. A poor training response will impact their championship performance. We shall look at two areas of anatomy subject to injury in aquatic athletes.
Keywords: Swimmers, shoulder, knee, anatomy

1 Overview

1.1 The shoulder

The shoulder is an intrinsically unstable joint with a large humeral head against a flat dish glenoid labrum surrounded by a capsule. Primary stability of the joint is the responsibility of condensations of the joint capsule called glenohumeral ligaments. These have been identified in the anterior capsule and recently there has been published documentation of condensations, although less well defined, within the posterior capsule, that suggests ligamentous structures. [2,3] The rotator cuff muscular investment is the secondary line of stability. Its primary responsibility being motion of the glenohumeral joint. Four groups of muscles are operating: Internal rotation:subscapularis, abduction: supraspinatus, external rotation:infraspinatus and teres minor, and adduction a combination of subscapularis and infraspinatus. A more superficial muscular layer attaching about the shoulder also provides motion, stability, and precision positioning. No amount of intrinsic strength of the external muscular investment seems able to prevent subluxation or dislocation of the shoulder joint if the primary capsular restraints are too lax.

Propulsive force in swimming is largely generated by the arms with the legs adding stabilization as well as propulsive force. [4] The shoulder joint is subject to a variety of repetitive microtrauma or over-use syndromes. [5,6] Not all swimmers under similar training load conditions will develop significant interfering shoulder complaints. [7] Most will escape any problems. The reason for this is likely multi-factorial, and, therefore, it is impossible to assign any single cause to the global problem of shoulder pain in swimmers. There is no truly definable entity called "swimmer's shoulder" but rather several problems in and about the shoulder may result in complaints of pain.

Because of the length of the lever-arm from the hand propeller to the shoulder, significant torque and shear forces occur at the glenohumeral joint surface. [4,8] Fine wire EMG studies show the external rotators, infraspinatus and teres minor, to have only a minor role during the swimming stroke. [9] It has been postulated that these muscles are overshadowed in their development by the more powerful swimming muscles, the adductors and internal rotators, that are constantly being trained. [10] We evaluated shoulder muscular adaptations in swimmers and water polo players and demonstrated changes in the rotator cuff force couples similar to those seen and documented in baseball pitchers. [11,12,13] These normal adaptive changes were predictable based on the mechanics of swimming and the EMG studies previously noted. [4,10] There appears to be an adaptive shift in the torque ratios of abduction:adduction and internal:external rotation towards the favor of adduction and internal rotation. [12,13] In an intrinsically stable shoulder joint, these adaptations seem well tolerated and therefore do not contribute to symptoms. However, in the individual with an unstable shoulder joint, the external rotators will be given extra responsibility to restrain any anterior subluxation which would occur during the press and insweep phases of the stroke. [10] This can lead to over use, inflammation and fatigue which may account for the common posterior pain in the individual with anterior subluxation.

A group of related studies assessed the torque production of the rotator cuff of swimmers and polo players and then tested a remedial program of specific exercise. Three consecutive studies were done. The first, involved senior and elite male competitive swimming athletes, [12] the second, elite water polo players, [13] and each were compared to college age controls. To assess the effect of the remedial exercise program, a group of NCAA Division III competitive swimmers were assigned to exercise vs. non exercise groups. They participated in a 12 week protocol to assess the effect of a specific exercise program on rotator cuff muscle torque development during a normal collegiate training cycle. [17]

Each subject was tested on the Cybex II Isokinetic Dynamometer for shoulder torque production during: internal rotation, external rotation, abduction and adduction at speeds of 30 and 180 degrees per second. The exercise protocol consisted of 5 exercises: 1) a direct lateral abduction exercise with a free weight, 2) this exercise isolated the supraspinatus muscle by holding the free weight with the thumb rotated towards the floor, then abducting in a plane 45 degrees forward of the frontal plane, 3) external rotation by lying in the lateral decubitus position with the arm adducted at the side and rotating 90° outward, 4) standard biceps curls in the frontal plane, and 5) designed for lower trapezius and scapula stabilization involved seated dips. A protocol was developed for all 5 exercises which included a recommended starting weight, suggested repetitions and numbers of sets for each exercise, a resistance increase protocol, and an ultimate resistance goal.

Table 1. Sample Exercise Protocol For Collegiate Male Swimmers

Exer #	Start Wt lbs (*)	Reps	# Sets	Wt Change	Wt Goal
1	10	20	3	2 lbs/2 wks	20
2	5	20	3	4 lbs/2 wks	15
3	4	20	3	4 lbs/2 wks	24
4	10	20	3	4 lbs/2 wks	30
5	10	20	1	+ 4/2 wks	30

* note, the start weight choosen should allow the performance of the full set prescribed

In adduction and abduction, the swimmers and polo players developed significantly greater torque than the controls in both arms and speeds. They also demonstrated significantly higher ratios resulting from a greater increase in torque development by the adductors compared to the abductors. [12,13]

In external and internal rotation, the swimmers and polo players developed significantly greater torque than controls in most comparisons. The ratios were significantly lower than controls for both arms and speeds. This resulted from a relative increase in torque production by the internal rotators compared to the external rotators. [12,13]

Statistical analysis of the torque values and ratios for the two groups of athletes in the remedial exercise study identified no significant differences but definite trends for most measurements. [14] We do believe that such a remedial program is of benefit and have used it clinically with satisfactory results.   There may methodological reasons for the non-significant results of this pilot study including small study group numbers, short study duration, and infrequent exercise bouts. This needs further evaluation. (28)

The shoulder and arm are neurologically represented by the cervical roots that coalesce into the brachial plexus and feed the entire upper extremity. Thus, the referred pain patterns that often accompany intrinsic disease of the cervical spine will have representation in the neck and upper extremity. The shoulder area is supplied by the C5 and C6 nerve roots, both from a sensory and motor aspect. Thus, cervical root dysfunction from tumor encroachment, herniated intervertebral disk or neuroforaminal stenosis from bony overgrowth may result in symptoms in and about the shoulder and upper arm. Similarly, tumors within the apex area of the lung, i.e., Pancoast tumor, by virtue of its proximity to the brachial plexus and impact on the sympathetic nervous system may result in shoulder area referred pain patterns and may also be accompanied by sympathetic dysfunction such as Horner's syndrome. A combination of neurologic and vascular problems may also manifest themselves in shoulder complaints, the most common of these being lumped as the thoracic outlet syndrome. This may result from impingement of the main vascular supply and/or brachial plexus on the first rib or scalene muscles as they exit the upper thorax and neck area and enter the arm. Axillary vein thrombosis may occure in the overhead athlete. The effects are prolongued and preclude return to vigorous sports in most cases. [25] Any thorough assessment of shoulder and upper extremity complaints, should include a neurologic examination of the upper extremity, a vascular assessment by various maneuvers such as the Adsen's test, and an evaluation of the lung apex by special radiographic views.

The acromioclavicular joint may undergo degenerative changes, develop synovitis, or damage to the meniscus like structure within the joint by a variety of activities. Shoulder separation can result from a direct blow to the point of the shoulder commonly seen during wrestling or football. This joint is often damaged as a consequence of high resistance weight training. This results in narrowing of the joint space, sclerosis of adjacent bone, erosions and, not uncommonly, osteophytes which may encroach on the subacromial space.

True glenohumeral arthritis is not common in the young athletic population but may be seen in the Masters group. This may result from a prior injury, either fracture or chronic shoulder instability. This can also occur late in the patient with a chronic massive disruption of the rotator cuff and is known as cuff arthropathy. In the young, inflammatory arthritic conditions, like rheumatoid arthritis, can involve the shoulder joint and result in its destruction.

It has become increasingly evident that glenohumeral instability is a final common denominator in many of the diverse diagnoses about the shoulder, including: tear of the glenoid labrum,[15] subacromial bursitis and rotator cuff tendinitis associated with impingement syndrome. [16] Anterior directional instability, either subluxation or frank dislocation, has long been recognized; it is now known that instability in other directions is also important and must be carefully assessed. [17] The overhead athlete is particularly vulnerable to developing multi-directional instability in which the glenohumeral joint may be subluxing or dislocating anteriorly, inferiorly, posteriorly and, to some extent, superiorly.

Thus, there may be some relationship, then, between instability and rotator cuff impingement syndrome. Here, a superior rising humeral head, as a consequence of a lax inferior joint capsule, produces compression of the supraspinatus tendon between the humeral head and the under surface of the acromial arch. This results in chronic abrasion and damage to the rotator cuff that leads to tendinitis of the supraspinatus and biceps tendons which are intimately juxta-positioned in the anterior superior aspect of the rotator cuff. Merely treating the symptoms of tendinitis may not provide a longstanding resolution of the problem if the underlying basic cause is instability. Many patients who have shoulder instability also manifest other signs of increased upper extremity laxity such as hyperextension of the elbows, laxity of the wrist joint, hyperextension of the metacarpal phalangeal joints and the ability to bring the tip of the thumb against the forearm in the wrist flexed position. Shoulder instability signs may be subtle but should be suspect whenever the patient complains of pain with sleeping, lifting heavy objects, positioning the arm in extremes of attitude, and performing such activities as push ups, pushing a door or reaching out to the side with an extended elbow. It is important to take a thorough functional history identifying those particular activities and positions where problems occur. Is there is evidence of noise or popping associated with the index activities? Does the patient feel apprehension in performing these activities or perceive the uneasiness of instability often described as feeling loose, lax or "going out"? A high index suspicion is needed in the early stages when the signs may be quite subtle and can only brought out by pointed questioning, discreet physical examination and even the necessity for an examination under anesthesia.

Another significant malady with resultant pain and restricted range of motion that not uncommonly is associated with a prior history of trivial trauma is adhesive capsulitis. A poorly understood, but relatively common, entity, it results in loss of range of motion of the shoulder. The capsule becomes contracted, capturing the joint, and resulting in significant loss of range of motion and disabling pain. It is not unusual, in a sequential fashion, to involve both shoulders. Treatment is prolonged and painful and requires a significant investment of time and energy by the patient, physician, and physical therapist. A daily exercise/stretching program is mandatory. Without treatment, the patient may be quite miserable for an extended period of time, often seeing an eventual spontaneous resolution of the process in 2-3 years. By instituting a vigorous, supervised therapy program, resolution of the process can often be accomplished in the 6 to 9 month time frame. For the patient who is unresponsive to treatment, distension of the joint capsule by infusion of fluid and local anesthetic followed by a manipulation, with or without general anesthesia, will often be helpful in speeding up the process of recovery of range of motion and diminution of disabling pain.

Chronic tendinitis of the rotator cuff from years of abuse may eventually weaken the cuff to the point that it will disrupt spontaneously or as a consequence of trivial trauma. The torn cuff retracts, exposing the humeral head which may rise up under the acromial arch. Pain is common. Weakness in shoulder abduction is pathognomonic. Atrophy of the supraspinatus muscle mass may result. While simple neglect may be a reasonable alternative for the sedentary elderly patient, most active patients of any age will be disabled and will require surgical repair of the disrupted cuff.

Treatment for most of the over-use inflammatory conditions in and about the shoulder consist of rest, non steroid anti-inflammatories, local heat and ice combinations, therapeutic stretching and rotator cuff muscle strengthening protocols. The use of selective injection techniques with anesthetic or in combination with corticosteroid may be helpful for both diagnosis and therapy. There is the potential that repeated injections of corticosteroid in and about tendinous structures may result in tendon weakening and delayed rupture. Some measure of rest and reduction in the index activity is indicated for these problems. For the variety of significant painful syndromes that do not respond to non operative treatment, a number of successful surgical interventions are available. In the case of subacromial impingement syndrome and rotator cuff tendinitis. Arthroscopic assisted techniques have been developed and have demonstrated efficacy matching the results of open surgical procedures yet halving the recovery time. [18] Degenerative problems of the acromioclavicular joint have been traditionally treated by surgical resection of the distal end of the clavicle. These techniques are also amenable to arthroscopic assisted techniques. [19]

Rotator cuff pathology often requires surgical intervention. While little can be accomplished arthroscopically for most patients with significant rotator cuff tears, simple debridement of tears in the elderly athlete may suffice for pain control. For most active patients who require strength, direct repair of the rotator cuff to the greater tubercle will be required. Attempts to accomplish this through mini incision arthroscopic assisted techniques may be applicable to small disruptions. More massive disruptions of the cuff are going to require an open technique. Stability of the shoulder joint must be reestablished through capsular reinforcement or tightening procedures. [17] A number of surgical procedures have been described, all having in common the tightening of the capsule ligamentous complex. Often there is some loss of extremes of range of motion in exchange for stability. Care must be taken in advising such procedures for the aquatic athlete who requires a significant range of motion for efficient execution. After such a stabilizing procedure some decrease in athletic performance might be anticipated.

In regards arthritic involvement of the glenohumeral joint, few options are available and will either prosthetic replacement or fusion of the joint. The latter procedure will be required with a history of infection or the young laboring individual who requires forceful use of the shoulder girdle and in whom a total joint replacement would rapidly fail. Neither the total joint replacement or the fusion operation would be compatible with the level of function required for any significant overhead sports activities.

1.2 The Knee

The knee of the swimmer is not commonly injured, and the most prevalent group of swimmers complaining of knee problems are breast strokers. It has been identified that the position of the knee center relative to the hip at the application of the extension and downward force in the breast stroke kick effects the amount of valgus stress applied to the medial collateral ligament and capsule complex of the knee joint. [20]   Those studies identified that the optimum initiation position for the kick is with the knee and hip centers aligned. If a wider or more narrowed position of the knee centers relative to the hips is selected, both result in increased strain on the medial knee joint. In the immature individual with open growth plates, this repetitive stress can injure the tibial and/or femoral growth plates resulting in localized pain. In addition, the medial collateral ligament and knee capsular structures may be over-strained in a repetitive fashion resulting in micro damage and inflammation. Swelling, localized tenderness and pain associated with the power phase of the kick will be noted and prevent appropriate training.

The patellofemoral articulation relies on a number of factors for stability including the ligamentous retinaculum support, both its medial and lateral investments, which stabilize the patella in the patellofemoral groove. The groove is usually formed so that the profile of the lateral buttress is higher than the medial thus containing the patella and resisting its tendency to sublux in a lateral direction. A patient born with a low lateral buttress has a much higher potential for the patella to ride out in a lateral direction resulting in subluxation. A laterally placed patella tendon attachment site at the tibial tubercle increases the patellofemoral, or "Q" angle, resulting in a lateral thrusting vector to the patella as the quadriceps contracts to extend the knee. Weakness of the vastus medialis obliqus, either from injury or chronic pain inhibition, can decrease its effectiveness in maintaining central tracking of the patella. This syndrome is often associated with a proximally placed patella, or "patella alta". If the patella attachment of the vastus medialis muscle has been stretched from repeated previous injuries, thereby decreasing its effectiveness in restraining the patella, a lateral patella migration may result. It has been shown that uniform pressure on the articular surface of the patella within the patellofemoral groove is important in maintaining its articular cartilage as it has no intrinsic blood supply. Cartilage nutrition is gained from the synovial joint fluid, and it relies upon diffusion and a gel pumping mechanisms to nourish the chondrocytes which are trapped within the hyaline cartilage matrix. Poor tracking of the patella, as a consequence of the above cited mechanisms, may thus lead to degeneration of the articular cartilage of the patella, called "chondromalacia". Decreased pressure on the medial facet because of lateral riding of the patella results in painful chondromalacia on the inferior medial facet of the patella. Patellofemoral instability is catastrophic for a breast stroke swimmer. In frank dislocation, surgery to realign the patella mechanism will be necessary for the athlete to continue practicing and competing. On the other hand, subluxation or mal-tracking of the patella may respond to a decrease in activity and retraining of the vastus medialis obliqus muscle through specific exercises. In addition, stretching of the quadriceps is helpful to reduce contracture which could increase the compressive forces on the damaged patella. The use of measures such as the McConnell taping techniques which are designed to decrease the lateral thrusting of the patella and re-coordinate the firing of vastus medialis in terminal extension may be helpful. [21]

Reactive inflammation of the patella tendon at the tibial tubercle attachment in the growing individual is not uncommon particularly when high loads are placed on this relatively soft attachment site durin running, jumping, pleiometrics, hard kicking and forceful knee extensions in weight training activities. This results in local swelling and pain and has been clinically described as Osgood-Schlatter's Syndrome. In the mature athlete, a similar mechanism of microtrauma results in a painfil tendinitis commonly referred to a "jumper's knee". The apparent mechanism of injury here is overload of the fibrocartilaginous tendon junction. Microscopic disruption of the attachment site results in scarring, local inflammation and swelling. Catastrophic failure of this tendon can occur and therefore reduction in activity is advised for the individual with symptoms.

Disruption of the medial collateral ligament of the knee may occur if it is subjected to high valgus strain loads. This usually requires an external force to be applied to the knee. However, tearing of the medial collateral ligament may occur in water polo players using the eggbeater kick. This a significant and disabling injury often requiring surgical repair.

Muscle injuries of the thigh are not uncommon. Muscle tears have occurred in elite level breast strokers. Excessive forces generated by legs built to high levels of muscle strength, can be sufficient to tear muscle, especially during eccentric contraction. Hamstring or adductor muscle disruption would preclude any significant participation in competitive swimming. The concern about such muscle injuries is that the resultant scarring and healing process may render the unit less compliant and therefore more subject to re-injury under future high load circumstances.

Damage to the fibrocartilage meniscus of the knee can occur during torquing and extension stress if the posterior portion of the meniscus is caught between the tibial and femoral joint surfaces. Tearing of the meniscus tissue results in a free edge that may be more easily trapped between the joint surfaces during bending and twisting type of activities. This will cause pain, often a snapping sensation, and, if the fragment is sufficiently large, locking of the joint. This can only be managed by arthroscopic repair or debridement of the damaged meniscus. Which technique is used is determined by the extent of the tear and its location within the body of the meniscus. Degenerative arthritis in the knee of the Masters Swimmer may be encountered. High stress loads placed on such a knee may result in complaints that preclude forceful kicking such as required in the breast stroke technique. Degenerative tearing of the meniscus in the arthritic knee is not uncommon and this would increase complaints. It seems that such knees tolerate the freestyle kicking mechanism better than that of breast stroke.

2 Summary

Thus, I believe medicine has much to offer the recreational or competitive aquatic athlete. Injury prevention is important and is supported by experience and research into injury mechanisms and causation factors. Quick identification of a correct diagnosis can allow the implementation of proper treatment and a more rapid return to full training capacity. Research can identify causation factors, faulty training methodologies and biomechanical facets which may promote injury. With this information and these tools, medicine can assist the coach in his responsibility to safely shepherd the athlete through the training phases to a maximum championship performance.

3 References

1. Clark K.S., Buckley W.E.(1980) Woman's injuries in collegiate sports. *Am. J. Sports Med.*, Vol. 8, pp. 187-191.
2. Turkel, S.J., Panio, M,W., Marshall, J.L., et al. (1981) Stabilizing mechanisms preventing anterior dislocation of the glenohumeral joint. *J. Bone Joint Surg.*, Vol. 63A. pp. 1208-1217.
3. Schwartz, R.E., O'Brien, S.J., Warren, R.F., et al. (1988) Capsular restraints to anterior-posterior motion of the shoulder. *Orthop. Trans.*, Vol. 12. pp. 277.
4. Schleihauf, R.E., Grey, L., DeRose, J. (1983) Three-dimensional analysis of hand propulsion in the front crawl stroke., (ed. A.P. Hollanger, P.A. Huijung, deGroot, G), *Biomechanics and Medicine in Swimming*, International Series on Sports Sciences, Vol.14, pp. 173-183, Human Kinetics Pub., Inc., Champaigne, Illinois.
5. McMaster, W.C., (1986) Painful shoulder in swimmers: a diagnostic challenge. *Phys. Sports Med.*, Vol.14. No.12, pp. 108-122.

6.   McMaster, W.C., Troup, J.P. (1993) A survey of interfering shoulder pain in United States competitive swimmers. *Am. J. Sports Med.,* Vol. 21, pp. 67-70.

7.   Fowler, P. (1979) Symposium: Swimmers problems. *Am. J. Sports Med.,* Vol. 7, pp. 141-142.

8.   Schleihauf, R. (1986) Swimming skill:A review of basic theory. *J. Swim. Res.,* Vol 2, pp. 11-20.

9.   Nuber, G.W., Jobe, F.W., Perry, J., Noynes, D.R., Antonellli D. (1986) Fine wire electromyography analysis of muscles of the shoulder during swimming. *Am. J. Sports Med.,* Vol 14. pp. 7-11.

10.   Fowler, P.J. (1988) Shoulder injuries in the mature athlete, *Adv. Sports Med.Fitness,* Vol 1. pp. 225-238.

11.   Aldernick, G.J., Kuck, D.J. (1986) Isokinetic shoulder strength of high school and college-aged pitchers. *J. Orthop. Sports Phys. Ther.,* Vol 7. pp. l63:l72.

12.   McMaster, W.C., Long, S., Caiozzo, V. (1991) Isokinetic torque imbalances in the rotator cuff of the elite water polo player. *Am. J. Sports Med.,* Vol 19. pp. 72-75.

13.   McMaster, W.C., Long, S., Caiozzo, V. (1992) Shoulder torque changes in the swimming athlete. *Am. J. Sports Med.,* Vol.20   pp. 323-327.

14.   McMaster, W.C. Assessment of the rotator cuff and a remedial exercise program for the aquatic athlete. *Medicine and Sports Science,* vol 39, S. Karger AG Pub. Basel, to be published 1994.

15.   McMaster, W.C. (1986) Glenoid labrum tears in swimmers: a cause of shoulder pain. *Am. J. Sports Med.,* Vol.14, pp. 383-387.

16.   Tibone, J.E., Jobe, F.W., Kerlan, R.K., et al. (1985)   Shoulder   impingement syndrome in athletes treated by an anterior acromioplasty. Clin. Orthop. Rel. Res. Vol. 198, pp.134-140.

17.   Neer, C.S., Foster, CR. (1980) Inferior capsular shift for involuntary and multidirectional instability of the shoulder. *J.Bone Joint Surg.,* Vol. 62A, pp. 897-908.

18.   Ellman, H. (1987) Arthroscopic subacromial decompression:an analysis of one to three year results. Arthroscopy, Vol. 3, pp. 173-181.

19.   Snyder, S., (1988) Arthroscopic acromioclavicular joint debridement and distal clavicle resection. *Tech. Orthop.,* Vol. 3, pp. 41-45.

20.   Kennedy, J. C., Hawkins, R. J.(1974) Breaststrokers knee. *Physician Sportsmed.,* Vol. 2., pp. 33-38.

21.   McConnell, J.,(1986) The management of chondromalacia patella:a long term solution. *Aust. J. Physiother.,* Vol. 32, pp. 215-223.

15 RELATIVE DISPLACEMENTS OF THE WRIST, ELBOW AND SHOULDER

V.J. DESCHODT, A.H. ROUARD and K.M. MONTEIL
Laboratoire de la Performance, C.R.I.S., U.F.R.A.P.S. Lyon France

Abstract

The purpose of this study was to identify the relative trajectories of the wrist and the elbow in reference to the shoulder displacement. 44 swimmers were filmed during the 100m freestyle races of the national Championships, using two videocameras. According to Schleihauf's method, the coordinates of the wrist, the elbow and the shoulder were obtained. The displacement of the wrist, elbow and shoulder were analysed with an external reference, in an antero-posterior axis. The wrist had a sinusoïdal path even if it had the same exit and entry points. During the middle of the time of the stroke cycle, this joint moved backward, and the population was very heterogeneous. For the elbow, the sinusoïdal path was flater. This joint moved never backward of the entry point. Its range was 0.96 m. The shoulder and the hip moved regulary and parallely during all the stroke. In reference to the shoulder displacement, the wrist seemed to slip backward during the middle time of the aquatic stroke, contrary to the elbow. It appeared a projection of the shoulder forward the elbow.

Keywords: Kinematic parameters, upper arm, trajectories, reference.

1 Introduction

Most of the studies were interested by the hand trajectory. In regard to the trajectories, Brown and Counsilman [1] have shown the sinusoïdal hand displacement in the 3 dimensions. For Maglischo et al. [2], the swimmers used lateral or vertical paths of their upper limb movement. All these studies considered the hand movement in reference to an external point. Maglischo [2] has mentioned that the slipping of the elbow would be the most serious mistake in swimming. To study this parameter, this author has observed the joint in relation to a reference on the swimmer himself, like the hip, to see how moves the joint in regard to this other. To show how a body moves in respect to the hand, Barthels [5] have used the analogy of a swimmer grabbing an underwater handle that was fixed to prevent it from moving backward as the hand pulls on it. According to these authors, it seemed that the hand did not move under the body but rather the body moves over the hands. For Counsilman [3], the displacement of the hand must be observed graphically in relation to the body. Counsilman [6] conclued that it would be possible and "also probable that there are some poor swimmers who accelerate their hands too greatly, thus "slipping" them though water.". In the same way, working about the division of swimming stroke into phases based upon kinematic parameters, Wiegand and al. [7] have suggested that the propulsion could be created mainly if the swimmer's hand moves faster backward than the body. That was the condition for the propulsive phase. To find this conclusion, these authors have made the difference between the relative horizontal velocity of the wrist joint movement and the hip joint velocity. Hay J.G. et al. [8] have studied the trunk roll in relation to hand pattern. They said that the swimmer must move the arm laterally relative to trunk.

The purpose of our study was to identify the relative trajectories of the wrist and the elbow with the shoulder as reference, and of the wrist with the elbow as reference. These relative displacements would be confronted with the real displacement of the joints, in relation to an external reference in an antero-posterior axis in order to determine if the overlapping of the joints resulted from the forward projection of the shoulder and/or of the slipping backward movement of the elbow and/or of the hand.

2 Protocol and measurements

44 swimmers have participated to this study. Their performance level and their anthropometrics data were reported in table 1.

Table 1: Characteristics of the population (N=44)

Parameters	Mean	Standard deviation	Range
Weight (kg)	78.94	15.02	27.2
Height (cm)	1.847	0.11	0.161
Age (years)	21.4	6.29	11
Performance in 100m races (s)	51.02	4.42	7.18

The swimmers have been filmed with 2 video cameras (30 Hz) during the 100 m freestyle races in National Championships. The two cameras were fixed in the extremity of the pool in underwater boxes (60 cm depth), and formed a right angle (90°) between themselves.

According to Schleihauf's software, a upper arm stroke of each swimmer has been digitized. One cycle was defined by the hand entry to the same hand exit. Five points (4 joints (wrist, elbow, shoulder and hip), and one point of external reference have been digitized. The 4 joints have been selected because of their specificity in the aquatic movement in freestyle. The external reference was the same point for all the frames. After the digitalisation, all the raw data have been smoothed with the Butterworth filter (function 3). We obtained the coordinates of all the points on the stroke, in an antero-posterior axis in reference to an external point. In the figure 1a, we can observe the wrist trajectory with an external reference.

In a second point, we have taken the shoulder as a reference point to express the relative displacement of the elbow and the wrist in the antero-posterior plan (Fig.1b). To obtain these relative displacements of the wrist and the elbow, we have subtracted the coordinates of the shoulder to the coordinates of the wrist or the elbow, frame by frame for all the stroke:

Relative displacement of the wrist = shoulder coordinates (t_j)- wrist coordinates (t_j)

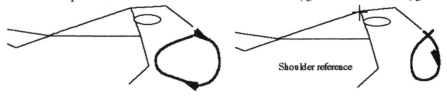

Shoulder reference

$+$ External reference

Fig.1. Wrist trajectories with an external reference and with the shoulder as reference

3 Results

The mean displacements of the joints (wrist, elbow, shoulder and hip) with an external reference in the horizontal axis have been observed. In the vertical axis, the displacement of each joint (m) have been noted. The value of the position of the joint at its entry in the water was represented by the 0 value. If this joint move forward in regard to this initial point, the displacement value will be positive. On the other hand, when the joint move backward, the value will be negative.

Table 2. Range and standard deviation of all parameters

Parameters	Range	Standard deviation	Maxi.	Mini
Wrist (m)	0.75	0.25	0.4	-0.65
Elbow (m)	0.96	0.28	0.96	0
Shoulder (m)	1.59	0.39	1.59	0

A sinusoïdal path of the wrist displacement in an antero-posterior axis has been noted (Fig 2). The wrist moved forward up to 29.63 % of the total cycle, then backward up to 77.77 % of the stroke. This two points have been defined as the maximal and the minimal values of the coordinates. The point the most forward of the trajectory have been represented by the maximal value of the coordinates. On the other hand, the point the most backwards of the trajectory was represented by the minimal value of the coordinates. The wrist overcrossed backward the entry point at 55.55 % (0.458 s (0.21 s)) of the total cycle, in regard to an antero-posterior axis. The range (difference between the maximal value of the coordinates and the minimal value) on the total cycle was 0.75 m (0.25 m) (Table 2). The wrist went out of the water at the same point of its entry, but during the cycle, this joint did not stay fixed. A positive relation (r=0.73) was observed between the hip velocity and the range of the wrist on the total cycle. Greater would be the range of the wrist trajectory, i.e., more the sinusoïdal length would be important, better would be the performance.

As for the wrist, a trajectory with a sinusoïdal tendancy was observed for the elbow, but flater than the first joint (Fig.2). The elbow was moving first forward up to 40.74% of the cycle, then backward up to 70.37 %. Contrary to the wrist, the maximal and minimal values were at the beginning and at the end of the aquatic stroke. The elbow did not move backward to the entry point. The range of this joint was 0.96m (0.28 m) (Table 2). Thus, the elbow was going out of the water 0.96m forward of the entry point. A relation (r=0.75) has been noted between the range of the elbow and the hip velocity. More the elbow came out of the water forward, better would be the performance. The shoulder and the hip (Fig.2) moved regulary and parallely during the aquatic stroke in regard to the antero-posterior axis. The range was 1.59 m (0.39 m) for the shoulder and 1.79 m (0.49 m) for the hip (Table 2). The shoulder was going out of the water 1.59 m forward of the entry point, and the hip 1.79 m forward.

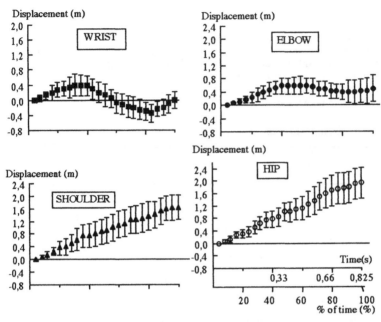

Fig. 2 Horizontal displacement of the different joints during the cycle for all the swimmers (N=44)

The ratio between the standard deviation and the range for each frame of the aquatic part of the cycle and for each joint were calculated (Fig 3). The greatest dispersion between the subjects was observed for the wrist joint, more especially during the middle of the time of the stroke. The subjects were more homogeneous for the elbow, shoulder and hip joints than for the wrist. The path of the wrist displacement seemed to have a great importance in regard to the others.

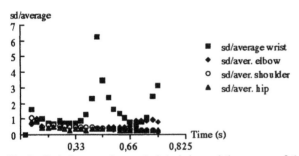

Fig. 3. Ratio between the standard deviation and the average of the horizontal displacement of the different joints for all the subjects.

The wrist and the elbow displacements in reference to the shoulder displacement, and the wrist displacement in reference to the elbow displacement have been represented (Fig 4). When the values of the relative coordinates of the joints were negative, that shown the first joint was forward the second. When this relative coordinates were 0, the two joints were in the same lines in regard to an antero-posterior axis. And when this coordinates were positive, the first joint were backward the second. A comparison between the relative displacement and the displacement with an external reference have been made to observe which joint slipped backward of the other, or conversely which was projected forward the second.

At the beginning of the aquatic stroke, the relative coordinates of the wrist in regard to the shoulder did not vary : the distance between the wrist and the shoulder did not change. At 20% of the cycle, the relative coordinates seemed to increase. The wrist came closer to the shoulder. At the same time the wrist moved backward with an external reference, whereas the shoulder moved always forward. The wrist was slipping backward the shoulder. It moved backward the shoulder at 68 % of the total cycle (0.51 s (0.07 s) (Table 3). After this instant, the wrist was moving away from the shoulder. A significative and positive relation (r=0.87) between the instant when the wrist overcrossed backward the shoulder and the hip velocity was observed. A high level of performance would be linked to a later slipping of the hand backward the shoulder.

Table 3. Mean and standard deviation of the relative time of the joints

Parameters	Mean	Standard deviation
Time wrist/shoulder (s)	0.51	0.07
Time shoulder/elbow (s)	0.47	0.08
Time elbow/wrist (s)	0.458	0.19
Hip velocity (m.s^{-1})	2.23	0.51

The relative displacement of the elbow in reference to the shoulder displacement (Fig. 4) varied during the cycle, but less than the wrist. During 32 % of the cycle, the elbow and the shoulder stayed in the same distance. With an external reference, the elbow stayed fixed during this part of the stroke. Then the relative coordinates seemed to increas, the elbow and the shoulder came closer, to be on the same line at 56 % (0.47 s (0.08 s)) (Table 3) of the total cycle. The elbow has a tendancy to stay fixed, whereas the shoulder was moving forward. In this case, a forward projection of the shoulder has been shown. A positive relation (r=0.65) between the time when the shoulder overcrossed forward the elbow and the hip velocity was pointed out. This relation was less important than for the wrist one. The slipping of the wrist seemed more important in regard to the performance level than the shoulder projection forward the elbow.

The coordinates of the wrist in reference to the elbow have been observed (Fig. 3). This two joints seemed to stay at the same distance up to 24 % of the total cycle. Then the value of the relative coordinates increased: the two joints were in the same line at 72% of the total cycle (0.595 s (0.09 s) in regard to an antero-posterior axis (Table 3). Whereas the elbow seemed to stay fixed during this part of the movement, the wrist was moving backward. There was a slipping of the wrist in regard to the elbow joint.

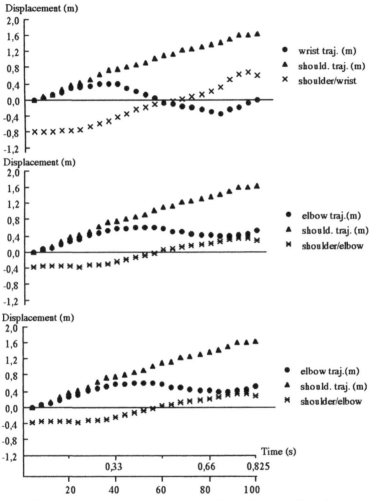

Fig. 4. Relative displacement of the wrist and the elbow with the shoulder reference, and of the wrist with the elbow reference, confronted to the horizontal displacement of this all joints.

4 Comments and conclusion

Contrary to many authors [1], [9], [4], who noted that the trunk overcrossed forward the hand, considering as fixed during the aquatic part, our study showed that the wrist had a sinusoïdal displacement in an antero-posterior axis. This joint moved forward in the first of the stroke, then backward up to the entry point, before to finish in the same point than the entry point. On the other words, the wrist had most variations during the stroke. A positive correlation coefficient between the range on the cycle of this joint and the hip velocity has been found : greater would be the difference between the maximal an the minimal value of the coordinates, better would be the hip velocity during the stroke. The elbow had a sinusoïdal path in the antero-poterior axis, but flater than the wrist. Thus, this joint did not move backward of the coordinate of the entry point. The relationships between the range of the elbow and the hip velocity showed that more the swimmers have a great amplitude of their elbow, better will be the hip velocity. The hip and the shoulder presented greater displacement than the elbow on the total aquatic stroke.

The greatest dispersion of the swimmer was observed for the wrist trajectory, especially during the middle of the time of the strocke, contrary to Maglischo [2] and Schleihauf [4], who have shown the importance of the downsweep phase in the aquatic part of the stroke.

In regard to the relative displacement, the wrist and the shoulder were in the same line in the antero-posterior axis at 68 % of the total cycle, after the slipping of the wrist backward to the entry point (55 %). The wrist had a tendancy to move back during the middle of the stroke with an external reference, whereas the shoulder continued to progress. On the other hand, no slipping of the elbow was observed. This joint was staying fixed during this part of movement, and it was the shoulder that moved forward. There was a projection of this joint forward the elbow, contrary to Maglischo's findings [2], who said that the elbow slipping would be the most serious error in swimming. The projection of the shoulder forward the elbow occured at the same time than the wrist slipping backward to the entry point.

5 References

1. Brown, R.M., Counsilman, J.E. (1971) The role of lift in propelling the swimmer. *J.M.Cooper (ed), Proceedings of the CIC Symposium on Biomechanics*, pp. 179-188, Indiana University.
2. Maglischo, C.W., Maglischo, E.W., Higgins, J., Hinricks, R., Luedtke, D., Schleihauf, R.E., Thayer, A. (1986) A biomechanical analysis of the 1984 U.S. Olympic Swimming Team: the distance freestylers. *Journal of Swimming Research*, Vol. 2, No. 3, pp. 12-16.
3. Counsilman, J.E. (1977) Pratical considerations of stroke mechanics. *Competitive Swimming Manual for Coaches and Swimmers*, Bloomington, Indiana, pp. 165.
4. Schleihauf, R.E. (1979) A hydrodynamic analysis of swimming propulsion. *J. Teraud and E.W. Bedingfield (eds), Swimming III, International Series on Sport Sciences*, Vol. 8, pp. 70-109, University Park Press, Baltimore.
5. Barthels, K.M. (1979) The mechanism for body propulsion in swimming. *J. Teraud and E.W. Bedingfield (eds), Swimming III, International Series on Sport Sciences*, Vol. 8, pp. 45-54, University Park Press, Baltimore.
6. Counsilman, J.E. (1981) Hand speed and acceleration. *Swimming Technique*, Vol. 18, No. 1, pp. 22-26.
7. Wiegand, K., Wuensch, D., Jaehnig, W. (1975) The division of swimming strokes into phases, based upon kinematic parameters. *L. Lewillie and J.P. Clarys (eds), Swimming II, International Series on Sport Sciences*, Vol. 2, pp. 161-166, University Park Press, Baltimore.
8. Hay, J.G., Liu, Q., Andrews, J.G. (1993) Body roll and handpath in freestyle swimming: a computer simulation study. *Journal of applied biomechanics*, Vol. 9, pp. 227-237.
9. Rackham, G.W. (1975) An analysis of arm propulsion in swimming. *L. Lewillie and J.P. Clarys (eds), Swimming II, International Series on Sport Sciences*, Vol. 2, pp. 174-179, University Park Press, Baltimore.

16 ENERGY EXPENDITURE DURING HIGH VOLUME SWIMMING TRAINING BY THE DOUBLY LABELED WATER (2H218O) METHOD

T.A. TRAPPE*, A. GASTALDELLI**, A.C. JOZSI*, J.P. TROUP* and R.R. WOLFE**

*U.S. Swimming, University of Colorado, Colorado Springs, USA.
**University of Texas, Metabolism Unit, Shriners Burns Institute, Galveston, TX USA

Abstract

The purpose of this study was to examine energy expenditure of swimmers during high volume training (17.5 ±1.0 km·day-1) using the doubly labeled water method. Five world-ranked female swimmers were administered a dose of 2H218O and monitored for nine days. Day five was a rest day from swimming training, while the other days consisted of two training sessions per day, lasting a total of five to six hours. Resting energy expenditure (REE) was measured on a non-training day. Isotopic enrichment and decay rates were determined from saliva samples taken when the subjects first awoke. Isotopic decay constants and total energy expenditure were calculated using the two-point method. Food quotients, calculated from three days of dietary recall, averaged 0.919 (range of 0.88 to 0.94) and were used to convert CO_2 production to total energy expenditure (TEE). There were no changes in total body weight or body composition (from skinfold measurements) over the measurement period and therefore, no changes in the pool size in which the isotopes were distributed. REE and TEE were 7.70 ± 0.49 and 20.81 ± 1.19 MJ·day-1, respectively. The results of this investigation describe the total energy demand of high volume swimming training, which may be used to address the dietary concerns of the competitive swimming athlete.

Keywords: swimming nutrition, resting energy expenditure

1 Introduction

There have been few investigations of energy expenditure during swimming training [□1-6□]. Further, these studies have only provided estimates of energy expenditure in the laboratory setting or during low volume swimming training. To our knowledge, no investigations have determined the total energy demands of completing the high volume training commonly encountered by swimmers training for top-level competition. The doubly labeled water (DLW) method has proven to be a valuable tool for determining energy cost in the field [□7-10□], and has recently been validated during swimming exercise [□6□]. Over the past two to three decades, training volume in competitive swimming has increased to over 20 km·day-1. Training of this duration can deplete the carbohydrate stores within the muscle [□3□], which may affect the swimmer's response to the training regimen [□3, 11□]. Therefore, if the swimmer is to optimally adapt to the training program, proper nutritional guidelines (i.e., amount and composition) must be available. Thus, the purpose of this investigation was to measure the total energy expenditure (TEE) during high volume swimming training by the DLW method.

2 Methods

2.1 Subjects
Five highly trained elite female swimmers (age: 19.7 ±1.0 yr; height: 178.3 ±2.0 cm; weight: 65.4 ±1.5 kg) served as subjects for this investigation. All subjects were informed of associated risks with the research and signed a consent form which adhered to the human subjects guidelines of the Institutional Review Board. All swimmers were members of United States Swimming's National Team and world-ranked in one or more of the competitive swimming distances.

2.2 Dosages, sampling protocol, and isotopic enrichment
A saliva sample (1-3 ml) for background enrichment was obtained from each subject at 1 p.m. on day 1. The isotopes were subsequently administered a weighed dose from a stock solution of 2H218O containing 10.15 atom percent excess 18O (Cambridge Isotope Laboratories, Cambridge, MA) and 99.9 atom percent excess 2H (ICON Services, Summit, NJ), which was determined from the dilution of an aliquot. The solution was given orally and the container was washed with 100 ml of tap water and also given to the subject.

Saliva samples (1-3 ml) were taken at each sampling period after at least 30 minutes of abstinence from fluid intake [□12, 13□]. Samples were collected soon after the subjects awoke at approximately 6 a.m. the morning after the loading dose was administered (day 2) and at this same time over the next 7 days (days 3-9). Samples were collected directly into glass vials, sealed to prevent evaporative fractionation, and immediately frozen until analysis.

H218O and 2H2O enrichment analysis was completed using an isotope ratio mass spectrometer (VG Isogas, Cheshire, England). The analyses of these isotopes have previously been described and completed in our laboratory [□14□].

2.3 Resting energy expenditure

Measurement of REE was determined on a non-training day (day five for 3 subjects and one week later for 2 subjects) with an MGM Metabolic Monitor (Utah Medical). The subjects rested for 6 hours after waking and were seated for 20 minutes prior to gas exchange analysis. A mask and non-rebreathing valve were used for the 10 minute collection period. No food was consumed 2 hours prior to REE determination. VO2 and VCO2 (ml·min-1) were determined during the 10 minute collection period and the equation of DeWeir was used to determine REE [□15□]:

$$REE \ (kcal·day-1) = (3.9·VO2 + 1.1·VCO2) · 1.44$$

and converted to MJ (1 MJ = 238.89 kcal).

2.4 Total energy expenditure

Carbon dioxide production (rCO2) was calculated using the two point method previously described by Schoeller, et al. [□16, 17□]. Food quotient (FQ) was calculated from dietary records taken on days 3, 4, and 6. Diet composition was analyzed using The Food Processor II (ESHA Research, Salem, OR) software. Macronutrient composition was determined for each diet and FQ was calculated [□18, 19□] and averaged over the three days.

TEE was calculated from rCO2 (liters·day-1) using the equation of DeWeir [□15□]:

$$TEE \ (kJ·day-1) = 4.63 · rCO2 + 16.49 · rCO2 / FQ.$$

2.5 Determination of body weight and composition

Body weight and composition were measured over the experimental period to monitor isotopic pool size and metabolizable energy stores. Semi-nude body weight was taken prior to the afternoon workout each day using a digital bathroom scale. Body composition was measured on days 2, 5, and 9 from the sum of six skinfold measurements: biceps, triceps, subscapularis, midaxillary, suprailliac, and abdomen using skinfold calipers.

2.6 Training sessions analysis

Total training volume was recorded for all subjects during the measurement period. There was no swim training performed on day 5 and the subjects were allowed to complete their choice of activities (following REE determination). The subjects trained in two groups: distance freestyle (FREE) and individual medley (IM). The FREE group completed the majority of the workout distance swimming freestyle, while the IM group completed the training using all four competitive strokes. One subject completed workouts in FREE for the first 4 days and IM for the last 4 days. Two subjects swam in the IM group and the other two subjects swam in the FREE group for the entire experimental period.

2.7 Statistical analysis

A one-way ANOVA with repeated measures over time was completed on daily body weight and body composition (skinfolds). A level of $p < 0.05$ was accepted as significant and all values are expressed as mean ± SE.

3 Results

Body mass (-0.04 ±0.24 kg) and composition did not change significantly over the nine days. Macronutrient composition of the diets averaged 11.5% protein, 68.1% carbohydrate, and 20.3% fat. The high carbohydrate composition of the diet was reflected in the food quotient, which averaged 0.92 ±0.008.

The mean distance completed by the FREE and IM groups (excluding day 5) were 18.2 ±1.2 km·day-1 and 16.8 ±1.1 km·day-1, respectively.

Resting energy expenditure was 7.70 ± 0.49 MJ ·day-1. Total energy expenditure of the subjects during the experimental period was 20.81 ±1.19 MJ ·day-1.

4 Discussion

This study was the first to determine the energy demands of high volume swimming training commonly encountered by top-level competitive swimmers by using the DLW method. Jones and Leitch [☐6☐] have also determined energy expenditure by the DLW method in swimming athletes, but the training volume completed in this study was much lower than in the current study. The DLW method has been validated during swimming exercise [6], during sedentary conditions [☐16, 20☐] and during high rates of energy expenditure [☐21, 22☐]; therefore, the DLW method appears to be a useful tool for measuring energy expenditure during swimming training.

The DLW method determines the average energy expenditure over the metabolic measurement period. The energy expenditure values for the subjects in this study included a day without swimming training, and actual values during the days of training may have been somewhat higher. If the rest day is factored out using the measured REE of each individual, the TEE for the days in which training was completed would have been 23.00 ±1.52 MJ·day-1.

Until now, there have been no investigations of the energy demands of swimming training for five to six hours per day in which distances of over 20 km·day-1 were completed. Previous investigations that have estimated the TEE during swimming training have examined distances less than 10 km·day-1. Costill et al. [☐3☐] have estimated the TEE of college males completing 9.0 km·day-1 to be 19.5 MJ·day-1. If the estimated swimming energy expenditure component is doubled in this investigation (since the current investigation completed twice that training volume), an estimate of TEE while swimming 18 km·day-1 would be approximately 28.9 MJ·day-1. Lamb et al. [☐23☐] found male swimmers training 9.2 km·day-1 were able to maintain energy balance while consuming 19.56 ±2.16 MJ·day-1. Additionally, Costill et al. [☐2, 11☐] estimated the energy expenditure of swimming 18 km·day-1 to be 18.8 MJ·day-1. The REE of the male swimmers is not included in this value; therefore, the TEE would be somewhat higher and consistent with the values observed in the current study.

Few studies have actually investigated energy expenditure in females swimmers. However, it is recognized that female swimmers are more economical than male swimmers [☐24☐]. Additionally, females are known to have lower REE than males. Therefore, if the above mentioned values are corrected for these differences, the TEE of the females in the current study are comparable.

In summary, this study gives a useful estimate of total energy expenditure of female swimmers completing a high training volume common in competitive swimming today. These data provide the coach and the athlete with guidelines for formulating an appropriate dietary regime that meets the energy requirements of elite training programs.

5 Acknowledgment

The authors would like to thank the subjects and United States Swimming's national team coaching staff for their cooperation during the data collection and Mrs. ??? for assistance with the isotope analysis.

6 References

1.   Beltz, J. D., D. L. Costill, R. Thomas, W. J. Fink, and J. P. Kirwan. (1988) Energy demands of interval training for competitive swimming. *Journal of Swimming Research*, Vol. 4, No. 3. pp. 5-9.

2.   Costill, D. L., J. Kovaleski, P. Porter, J. Kirwan, R. Fielding, and D. King. (1985) Energy expenditure during front crawl swimming: Predicting success in middle-distance events. *International Journal of Sports Medicine*, Vol. 6, No. 5. pp. 266-270.

3.   Costill, D. L., M. G. Flynn, J. P. Kirwan, J. A. Houmard, J. B. Mitchell, R. Thomas, and S. H. Park. (1988) Effects of repeated days of intensified training on muscle glycogen and swimming performance. *Medicine Science Sports and Exercise*, Vol. 20, No. 3. pp. 249-254.

4.   Jang, K. T., D. L. Costill, J. P. Kirwan, J. A. Houmard, J. B. Mitchell, and L. J. D'Acquisto. (1987) Energy balance in competitive swimmers and runners. *Journal of Swimming Research*, Vol. 3, No. 1. pp. 19-23.

5.   Vallieres, F. A., A. Tremblay, and L. S.-Jean. (1989) Study of the energy balance and the nutritional status of highly trained female swimmers. *Journal of Nutrition Research*, Vol. 9, No. 7. pp. 699-708.

6.   Jones, P. J., and C. A. Leitch. (1993) Validation of doubly labeled water for measurement of caloric expenditure in collegiate swimmers. *Journal of Applied Physiology*, Vol. 74, No. 6. pp. 2909-2914.

7.   DeLany, J. P., D. A. Schoeller, R. W. Hoyt, E. W. Askew, and M. A. Sharp. (1989) Field use of D218O to measure energy expenditure of soldiers at different energy intakes. *Journal of Applied Physiology*, Vol. 67, No. pp. 1922-1929.

8.   Hoyt, R. W., T. E. Jones, T. P. Stein, G. W. McAninch, H. R. Lieberman, E. W. Askew, and A. Cymerman. (1991) Doubly labeled water measurement of human energy expenditure during strenuous exercise. *Journal of Applied Physiology*, Vol. 71, No. 1. pp. 16-22.

9.   Westerterp, K. R., W. H. M. Saris, M. v. Es, and F. T. Hoor. (1986) Use of the doubly labeled water technique in humans during heavy sustained exercise. *Journal of Applied Physiology*, Vol. 61, No. 6. pp. 2162-2167.

10.   Westerterp, K. R., B. Kayser, F. Brouns, J. P. Herry, and W. H. M. Saris. (1992) Energy expenditure climbing Mt. Everest. *Journal of Applied Physiology*, Vol. 73, No. 5. pp. 1815-1819.

11.   Costill, D. L., R. Thomas, R. A. Roberls, D. Pascoe, C. Lambert, S. Barr, and W. J. Fink. (1991) Adaptations to swimming training: influence of training volume. *Medicine Science Sports and Exercise*, Vol. 23, No. pp. 371-377.

12.   Schoeller, D. A., W. Dietz, E. van Santen, and P. D. Klein. (1982) Validation of saliva sampling for total body water determination by H218O dilution. *American Journal of Clinical Nutrition*, Vol. 35, No. pp. 591-594.

13.   Drews, D., and T. P. Stein. (1992) Effect of bolus fluid intake on energy expenditure values as determined by the doubly labeled water method. *Journal of Applied Physiology*, Vol. 72, No. 1. pp. 82-86.

14.   Goran, M. I., E. J. Peters, D. N. Herndon, and R. R. Wolfe. (1990) Total energy expenditure in burned children using the doubly labeled water technique. *American Journal of Physiology*, Vol. 259, No. 22. pp. E576-E585.

15.   DeWeir, J. B. (1949) New methods for calculating metabolic rate with special reference to protein metabolism. *Journal of Physiology* (London), Vol. 109, No. pp. 1-9.

16.   Schoeller, D. A., E. Ravussin, Y. Schutz, K. J. Acheson, P. Baertschi, and E. Jequier. (1986) Energy expenditure by doubly labeled water: validation in humans and proposed calculation. *American Journal of Physiology*, Vol. 250, No. 19. pp. R823-R830.

17.   Schoeller, D. A., and P. B. Taylor. (1987) Precision of the doubly labeled water method using the two-point calculation. *Human Nutrition: Clinical Nutrition*, Vol. 41C, No. pp. 215-223.

18.   Black, A. E., A. M. Prentice, and W. A. Coward. (1986) Use of food quotients to predict respiratory quotients for the doubly labeled water method of measuring energy expenditure. *Human Nutrition: Clinical Nutrition*, Vol. 40C, No. pp. 381-391.

19.   Southgate, D. A. T., and J. V. G. A. Durnin. (1970) Calorie conversion factors. An experimental reassessment of the factors used in the calculation of the energy value of human diets. *British Journal of Nutrition*, Vol. 24, No. pp. 517-535.

20.   Schoeller, D. A., and P. Webb. (1984) Five day comparison of the doubly labeled water method with respiratory gas exchange. *American Journal of Clinical Nutrition*, Vol. 40, No. pp. 152-158.

21.   Schulz, L. O., S. Alger, I. Harper, J. H. Wilmore, and E. Ravussin. (1992) Energy expenditure of elite female runners measured by respiratory chamber and double labeled water. *Journal of Applied Physiology*, Vol. 72, No. 1. pp. 23-28.

22.   Westerterp, K. R., R. Brouns, W. H. M. Saris, and F. t. Hoor. (1988) Comparison of doubly labeled water with respirometry at low and high activity levels. *Journal of Applied Physiology*, Vol. 65, No. 1. pp. 53-56.

23.   Lamb, D. R., K. F. Rinehardt, R. L. Bartels, W. M. Sherman, and J. T. Snook. (1990) Dietary carbohydrate and intensity of interval swimming training. American Journal of Clinical Nutrition, Vol. 52, pp. 1058-1063.

24.   Chatard, J. C., J. M. Lavoie, and J. R. Lacour. (1991) Energy cost of front-crawl swimming in women. *European Journal of Applied Physiology*, Vol. 63, pp. 12-16.

17 SHOULDER MUSCLE TORQUE CHANGES OF ELITE GERMAN AGE GROUP SWIMMERS

J. HOLZ, H. BÖTHIG, E. HILLE and K.M. BRAUMANN
Orthopaedic Dep., Allgemeines Krankenhaus Hamburg-Barmbek; Olympic Training and Research Center Hamburg; University of Hamburg, Dept. of Sports Sciences, Germany

Abstract
The purpose of this prospective study was to determine if clinical changes [1,2,3,4,5] and shifts of muscle torque ratios typically found in adult athletes [6] can also be seen in elite age group swimmers and whether a functional dryland strength training effects subclinical changes which are associated with the sport specific stroke mechanism and the development of overuse-syndromes and sport injuries of the shoulder in the competitive swimmer.

After undergoing a initial specific orthopaedic test programme and an isokinetic muscular strength test 31 elite age group swimmers trained with a functional muscular strength-training and flexibility programme over the timeperiod of 18 month. The results were compared to controls (n=20).

The shoulder-strength testing was performed on the Cybex II dynamometer for external and internal rotation in two test positions and two different testing modes.

The initial results demonstrated a significant muscular dysbalance of the internal rotation muscles (IR) to the external rotation muscles (ER) in male and female age group swimmers. A ratio of 1:2,22-1:1,78 (45-56 %) ER/IR was found in swimmers. In the controls a ratio of 1:1,47 - 1:1,41 (68-71 %) was measured.

Initially 16 swimmers mentioned shoulder problems within the last two years of training. A clinical manifest shoulder joint instability could be proved in 22 swimmers.

At the end of the study the results showed a significant increase of the external rotation muscles (ER). The ratios of 1:1,47-1:1,35 (68-74 %) ER/IR were determined in the swimmers.

In the final clinical testing instability was still seen in eigth shoulders. A single athlete had suffered from shoulder problems.

Keywords: age group swimmers, functional muscular strength-training, isokinetic test, muscle torque ratio shift, sport specific stroke mechanism, swimmers' shoulder

1 Introduction

It is known that "swimmers' shoulder" is the most frequent musculoskeletal complaint in competitive swimming [2,3,4,5,6,7]. The reason is the sportspecific repetitive stroke mechanics [4,6], which leads to an overuse of the active muscular and ligamentary elements which are stabilising the glenohumeral joint. Clinical changes typically found in adult athletes can be discovered in age group swimmers already after a few years of training. These subclinical changes and general joint laxity in swimmers could cause the development of impingement-syndroms and sport injuries later in the career.

It is the hypothesis of this study that the incidence of swimmers' shoulder can be reduced by introducing a dryland strength training for the antagonist muscles of internal rotation to swimmers. A normal ratio of muscular strength [4] prevents joint translation and establishes a optimal dynamic joint movement through the range of motion, in order to avoid secondary impingement problems [7].

2 Methods

2.1 Subjects and performance characteristics
The subjects for the study were 16 male and 15 female elite age group swimmers (age: ☐ 15.3 years) of the same training centre. All of them were finalists of the German age group championships or within the full second of the eighth placed swimmer.

The controls were 20 same aged non-swimmers and non-overhead associated sports high school students.

2.2 Isokinetic testing
Each subject performed an isokinetic muscular strength test initially, after 2 and 18 month on a Cybex 6000 dynamometer (Lumex Inc., Ronkonkoma, NY) for torque production in the shoulder joint in two test positions for internal and external rotation [9,10]. The testing was performed on the left and right sides at 60°/s and 180°/s speed with five and twenty repetitions per set in 90° abduction and 90° forward flexion. A five minute lasting brake was taken in between the sets.

2.3 Clinical testing
A standardised examination of the shoulder for instability of the shoulder joint and inflammatory or structural changes of the rotatorcuff-muscles was performed at the beginning and at the end of the study.

2.4 Clinical history
A complex questionnaire was conducted initially and at the end of the study for pain location and injury history, for pain related training tasks and stroke patterns.

2.5 Remedial training programme

Over a training period of eigtheen month swimmers carried out a three step dry land strength and flexibility training for external rotating muscles in the shoulder [8,9,11, 12,13,14].

For the first three weeks the athletes trained only with isometric exercises within their normal warm up programme or weight training.

Starting in the fourth week isotonic exercises were introduced to the training using Therabands and rubber bands.

After six weeks weight exercises started on Pulley kit and "Schnell"-training-devices. Over the training season the percentage of external rotation exercises increased to about 30 % of the entire dry land weight training exercises.

3 Results

Initially 16 swimmers mentioned shoulder problems within the last two years of training. A clinical manifest shoulder joint instability could be proved in 22 swimmers. In the final clinical examination instability was still seen in 8 shoulders. A single athlete had suffered from shoulder problems.

Fig. 1. Clinical findings

Clinical findings	Number of athletes (initial)	Number of athletes (final)
Instability:		
- anterior	11	5
- posterior	1	none
- multidirectional	3	1
Hyperlaxity	7	3
Impingement	1	none
Normal shoulder	8	22

Fig. 2. History of pain

Complaint/pain	Counts (initial)	Counts (final)
During swimming	12	1
Without swimming	7	1
Recovery phase	10	0
Early pull through	3	0
Late pull through	10	1
Competition	2	0

Aerobic-endurance training	6	1
Anaerobic training	7	0
Paddles	7	1
Freestyle	11	1
Breaststroke	1	0
Butterfly	3	1
Backstroke	3	0

The initial results of the isokinetic testing demonstrated a significant muscular dysbalance [15,16] of the internal rotation muscles (IR) to the external rotation muscles (ER) of the shoulder in male and female age group swimmers.

Fig. 3. Initial isokinetic testing , values of external rotation . internal rotation

Testing mode	swimmers (male)	swimmers (female)	controls (male)	controls (female)
1. 90° forw. flexion	50 % (1:2)	45 % (1:2,22)	62 % (1:1,61)	66 % (1:1,52)
2. 90° abduction	56 % (1:1,79)	56 % (1:1,79)	74 % (1:1,35)	71 % (1:1,41)

The two following isokinetic retests were performed in the same mode as described (e.g. 2.2.) and documented the increase of strength values for the external rotation.

Fig. 4. Development of values of external rotation : internal rotation within 18 month, entire group

Testing mode	1. Test (initial)	2. Test (2 month)	3. Test (18 month)	total increase
1. 90° forw. flexion	47 % (1:2,13)	52 % (1:1,92)	63 % (1:1,59)	**34,0 %**
2. 90° abduction	56 % (1:1,79)	61 % (1:1,64)	74 % (1:1,35)	**32,1 %**

4 Discussion

This study has documented that the age group competitive swimming athlete develops clinical changes, pain syndromes and shifts in torque production for external : internal rotation in the shoulder [17].

After introducing a remedial strengthening programme of the external rotators for eighteen month normal values for shoulder torque ratios were determined and swim related shoulder pain were significantly reduced.

The results of this study indicate that a remedial dry land programme can have an effect on joint stability and on an ideal dynamic synchronised joint movement through the sport-specific activity of swimming.

It seems that a general hyper laxity frequently seen in swimmers and a torque ratio shift due to swim-specific stroke pattern [18] might potentiate joint translation in the glenohumeral joint which provokes instability related impingement.

It is described that the muscular and ligamentary structures obtain their final shape and function within puberty. A too early highly specified swim training will cause inadequate isolated muscle strengthening with the risk of unsynchronised joint movement and later in the career occurring overuse syndromes.

The aim of coaches and physicians should be to prevent those overuse syndromes in swimmers by introducing a remedial functional strengthening programme for the external rotators of the shoulder.

5 References

1. Ciullo, Jerome V.; Stevens, Gregory G. (1989), *The prevention and treatment of injuries to the shoulder in swimming*, Sports Medicine, Vol.7, 182-204

2. Ciullo, Jerome V. (1986), *Swimmer's Shoulder*, Clinics in Sports Medicine, Vol.5, No. 1

3. Fowler, Peter J. (1991), *Upper Extremity Swimming Injuries*, Chapter 40, Section 5, The Upper Extremity in sports medicine, James E. Nickolaus

4. Johnson, J.E.; Sim, F.H.; Scott, S.G. (1987), *Muscoloskeletal injuries in competitive swimmers*, Mayo Cinics Proc., Vol.62

5. McMaster, William C.; Troup, J. (1993), *A survey of interfering shoulder pain in United States competitive swimmers*, The American Journal of Sports Medicine, Vol.21, No.1, S. 67-70

6. McMaster, William C.; Long, Susan; Caiozzo,Vincent (1992), *Shoulder torque changes in the swimming athlete*, The American Journal of Sports Medicine, Vol.20, No.3

7. Jerosch, J.; Castro, W.H.M.; Sons, H.U. (1990), *Das sekundäre Impingement-Syndrom beim Sportler*, Orthopädische Klinik und Poliklinik Düsseldorf Sportverletzung und Sportschaden, Nr.4, 180-185, Georg Thieme Verlag

8. Burkhead, W.Z.; Rockwood, Ch.A. (1992), *Treatment of instability of the schoulder with an exercise programm*, The Journal of Bone and Joint Surgery, Vol.74-A; No.6

9.   Davies, George J. (1987), *A compendieum of isokinetics in clinical usage and rehabilitation techniques*, S & S Publishers, 1707 Jennifer Court, Onalaska, Wisconsin 54650

10. Seibert, G.; Verdonck, A.; Duesberg, F. (1991), *Isokinetische Systeme - Funktionsprüfung und Kalibrierung*, mt-Medizintechnik 111, Nr.5, S.165-172

11. Janda, David H.; Loubert, Peter (1991), *A preventative program focusing on the gelenohumeral joint*, Clinics in Sports Medicine, Vol.10, No.4

12. Penny, J.Norgrove; Smith, Clyde (1980), *The Prevention and Treatment of Swimmer's Shoulder*, Canadian Journal of Applied Sports Science, 5:3, 195-202

13. Shrode, L.W. (1994), *Treating shoulder impingement using the supraspinatus synchronization exercise*, Journal of Manipulative Physiological Therapeutics17, No.1, S. 43-53

14. Tittel. K. (1989), *Funktionell-anatomische und biomechanische Grundlagen für die Sicherung des "arthro-muskulären Gleichgewichts" im Sport*, Beitrag zur Erhöhung der Belastbarkeit bindegewebiger Strukturen, Bd.1, S.2-4

15. Habermeyer, Peter (1989), *Isokinetische Kräfte im Glenohumeralgelenk* Springer - Verlag, ISBN 3-540-51122-9

16. Ivey, Frank M.; Calhoun, Jason H.; Rusche, Ken et al. (1985), *Isokinetic testing of shoulder strength: Normal values*, Arch. Phys. Med. Rehabilitation, Vol.66

17. Ungerechts, Bodo; Bieder, A. (1992), *Muskelkraftungleichgewichte in der Schultermuskulatur jugendlicher Leistungsschwimmer* unpublished study, Olympiastützpunkt Hannover

18. Scovazzo, Mary L.; Browne, Anthony; Pink, Marilyn et.al. (1991), *The Painful Shoulder during Freestyle Swimming: An EMG and cinematographic analysis of twelve muscles*, The American Journal of Sports Medicine, Vol.19, No.6

PART FOUR

PHYSIOLOGICAL ASPECTS

18 METABOLIC DEMANDS FOR SWIMMING

S.W. TRAPPE

Human Performance Laboratory, Ball State University, Muncie, IN USA

Abstract
The majority of swimming events are less than 2 minutes in duration. During exercise bouts of this brief duration, anaerobic ATP production is the primary energy source for the active skeletal muscles. More importantly, the rate at which ATP is delivered also influences muscle contraction and in turn, swimming speed. Thus, it would appear that a large capacity for anaerobic energy production is beneficial for fast swimming. Information describing the anaerobic capacity reveals distinct differences between sprint and endurance trained athletes for both the capacity and the rate at which fuel is supplied to the contracting muscles during high-intensity exercise. This high glycolytic demand corresponds well with glycogen breakdown and glycolytic enzyme activities of the muscles when exercising at supramaximal intensities ($>100\%$ VO_2max). However, lactate alone appears to be a poor indicator of total anaerobic energy yield during high-intensity exercise. These data emphasize the importance of anaerobic energy release during swimming competition. Currently, the swimming community advocates volume overload training to produce optimal performances. Due to the high degree of muscle plasticity and physiological adaptability, coaches and athletes should be aware of the specific adaptations during this type of swimming training. Practical methods on the pool deck (a stopwatch) and proper nutritional guidelines can serve to gauge the effectiveness of their training plan on swimming speed.
Keywords: Anaerobic Capacity, Glycogen, Lactate, Metabolism.

1. Introduction

By most opinions, swimming is considered an endurance and power sport. This has made designing a swimming training program that will elicit the ideal metabolic adaptations for optimal swimming performance a challenging task. The intensity and volume of training generally employed during swimming practice stresses both the aerobic and anaerobic energy systems; however, anaerobic energy production is the major contributor during competition. This is further emphasized by the fact that more than 80% of competitive swimming events are less than 2 minutes in duration. Thus, a large anaerobic capacity may be a prerequisite for fast swimming. This presentation will begin with a brief overview on muscular adaptations from swim training, followed by the importance of anaerobic energy contribution during high-intensity exercise. In closing, practical applications along with unsolved issues will be presented.

2.   Muscular Adaptations

Endurance training induces major alterations in skeletal muscle and has been examined quite extensively [cf. 2, 3]. Experience has shown that the endurance capacity of an athlete is usually attained within the first 6-8 weeks of training and further gains in aerobic endurance are minimal. The high volume nature of swimming training also lends itself to numerous endurance attributes in the skeletal muscle. Most notably, there is a significant increase in the size and density of mitochondria, the aerobic powerhouse of the muscle cell [4]. Oxidative enzymes, such as citrate synthase have also been shown to increase during the course of a swim season [5]. However, the degree to which glycolytic enzyme concentrations are altered with swimming training is debatable. This is related to the relatively high capacity of the glycolytic system in less-trained individuals, and may actually be compromised with mild endurance activity.

The capillary vasculature within the muscle bed also increases dramatically following periods of high volume, high intensity training. This plays a paramount role in oxygen delivery to the tissues as well as the removal of carbon dioxide and the efflux of various metabolites from the muscle. In addition, blood volume increases with training [6], and when coupled with the increased capillary network, may allow for greater perfusion of the skeletal muscle during "all-out" swimming.

Swimming training also induces muscle hypertrophy which is mediated through structural adaptations in the muscle fibers. However, the degree of muscle hypertrophy greatly depends upon the type of training stimulus provided to the muscle fibers. The increase in muscle fiber size has been shown to be more pronounced in the type II muscle fibers with exercise training [7, 8]. Furthermore, these alterations have been suggested to be primarily related to increases in actin and myosin filaments, resulting in a greater number and size of myofibrils [9].

The contractile and mechanical properties of skeletal muscle have been shown to change with swimming training. This was examined using single muscle fibers from the human deltoid muscle during periods of heavy swim training [10]. There was no change in the force-velocity relationship or peak tension (P_0) in the different fiber types. However, a subsequent decrease in maximal shortening velocity (V_{max}) of type II fibers was observed. These alterations may have a direct impact upon the ability of skeletal muscle to generate tension. More importantly, if the contractile network is compromised with endurance training, it may be responsible for subpar swimming performances. More research is needed in this area to determine how the contractile machinery responds to different training modalities.

3.   Anaerobic Energy Yield

From the previous discussion, it is apparent that swim training significantly enhances the endurance potential of the muscle. However, the competition needs of swimming require the muscle to perform at the highest sustainable work rate for the duration of the event. In doing this, the glycolytic component of the muscle cells are placed under severe stress to

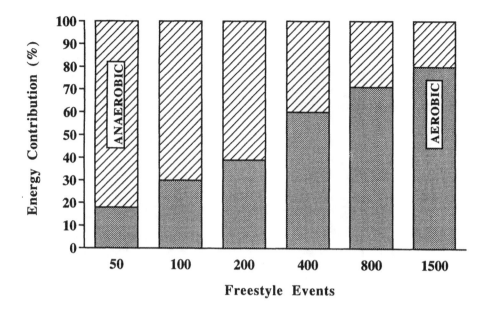

Figure 1. Relative energy contribution for freestyle swimming events.

produce ATP quickly. To help understand the anaerobic energy release and provide insight into the rate of anaerobic energy production, we examined the anaerobic capacity and skeletal muscle components in sprint and endurance trained athletes [11].

As noted in figure 1, the demands of the glycolytic system are greatest in events that range from 50 to 200 meters, resulting in a high rate of energy delivery to the contractile machinery of the muscles. This underscores the importance for an extremely high glycolytic energy yield in human skeletal muscle during swimming competition.

3.1 Whole-body oxygen deficit

Oxygen deficit measurements were made at 110% of VO_2max until volitional exhaustion. The anaerobic capacity (AC) was determined as the difference between the estimated total energy demand and the accumulated oxygen uptake [12, 13]. As shown in figure 2, the sprint subjects had a larger AC as compared with the endurance subjects.

To examine differences in anaerobic power production, the percent contribution over time was compared to the total anaerobic energy yield (figure 3). From this, it was obvious that the sprint athletes not only had a larger anaerobic tank, but they were also able to provide a greater sustained anaerobic energy supply during the entire exercise bout.

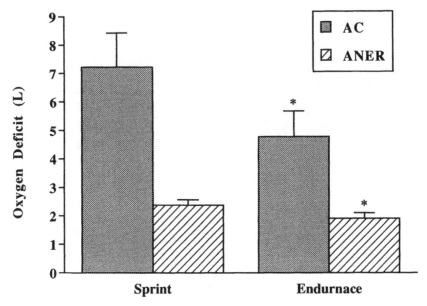

Figure 2. Mean values for anaerobic capacity (AC) and anaerobic energy release (ANER) at 30 sec from the oxygen deficit test. *p<0.05 = difference between sprint (n=6) and endurance (n=6) athletes.

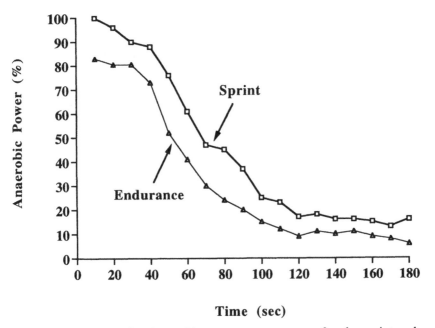

Figure 3.   Anaerobic power output curves for the sprint and endurance athletes. Data are expressed in 10 sec increments based on the total anaerobic capacity obtained during the deficit test.

Using a few calculations, the amount of power production in watts was determined. The sprint athletes generated a total of 1719 ± 132 watts compared with 1429 ± 146 watts by the endurance athletes. Calculations for theoretical anaerobic ATP production (6.5 mol ATP = 1 mol O_2) during the exercise bout suggests that the sprinters were able to produce substantially more ATP via anaerobic sources (7494 ± 561 vs. 6230 ± 611). This gives an indication of ATP turnover and reiterates the importance and ability of sprint trained athletes to rapidly provide high energy phosphates to the working muscle.

3.2 Glycolytic rate

In addition to the higher AC, the sprint athletes also demonstrated a higher anaerobic energy release (ANER) at 30 seconds (figure 2). The ANER has been shown by Medbo et al. [14] to reflect an enhanced rate of energy release of anaerobic sources in the working muscles. The sprinters had delivered 19.7% more energy via anaerobic sources at 30 seconds than the endurance group. While this is not a measure of anaerobic capacity, it is reflective of the rate of ATP turnover when placed under intense stress [15]. Although the sprint group did elicit a greater ANER at 30 seconds, it only represented 32.9% of their AC, whereas the endurance group's fractional utilization had reached 40.0% of their capacity. Thus, not only did the sprint group have a larger anaerobic capacity, they were also able to provide a greater amount of energy anaerobically while a greater reserve was available for subsequent power production.

Muscle biopsies were obtained from the vastus lateralis prior to and immediately following the exercise bout [16]. Muscle glycogen concentrations from the muscle homogenates are in Table 1. No differences in pre exercise muscle glycogen was observed between groups prior to the oxygen deficit test. However, post oxygen deficit test muscle glycogen was significantly (P<0.05) lower in the sprint group. Consequently, the sprinters utilized a greater (P<0.05) amount of glycogen during the exercise bout as compared with the endurance athletes. The amount of glycogen utilized was more than 2-fold greater in the sprint athletes. This suggests that the sprint group was able to provide a greater amount of ATP via glycolysis which helped account for the greater anaerobic energy release.

Table 1. Pre and post oxygen deficit test muscle glycogen concentrations and enzyme activity from the sprint and endurance trained athletes.

| Group | Muscle Glycogen Values | | | |
	Pre	Post	Δ	Phosphorylase
Sprint	124.4 ± 14.8	72.6 ± 3.8	51.8 ± 13.8	21.2 ± 2.5
Endurance	112.2 ± 15.6	88.1 ± 6.6*	24.1 ± 11.3*	9.6 ± 5.0*

*p<0.05 between groups. Muscle glycogen = mmol•kg^{-1} ww;
phosphorylase = μmol•g^{-1}•min^{-1}

3.3   Metabolic Controllers

A key process for glucose availability, is the conversion of glycogen to glycogen-1-phosphate, in which the catalytic rate is controlled, in part, by glycogen phosphorylase [17]. As a result, a high concentration of this enzyme (or other enzymes) may allow for a greater conversion rate, and a superior anaerobic energy delivery. The sprinters did demonstrate a greater ($p<0.05$) phosphorylase activity (table 1), which also revealed a strong relationship ($r=0.86$) to the total anaerobic energy yield. In contrast, citrate synthase activity was found to have a low relationship ($r=-0.47$) to the measured anaerobic capacity.

Lactate has also been implicated as a key regulator during high intensity exercise [18]. The production of lactate and its dissociation in the cytosol of the muscle cell to elicit free H^+ and significantly lower muscle pH has been shown have a profound impact upon fatigue and muscle performance [19]. In the present study, there were no differences in muscle or blood lactate concentrations after the exercise test. Since only absolute concentrations were measured with no a-v difference determinations it is difficult to ascertain why similar concentrations were found. However, several investigators [cf 20, 21] have concluded that lactate in the muscle and extra-cellular fluid together provide a relative contribution ranging from 67-78% of the total anaerobic production. On this basis, it would not be expected that lactate measurements accurately reflect the total anaerobic energy yield. Furthermore, differences in muscle perfusion may have contributed to a wide variation in lactate kinetics and their effect on the cellular environment.

4.   Practical Applications

There have been numerous nutritional investigations involving endurance capacity and intermittent, high intensity exercise. However, swimming represents a unique situation in that, over a two hour plus time period athletes engage in moderate to very intense exercise which places a large demand on the carbohydrate reservoir in the body. The majority of the training involves interval type work in a range of 80-120% of VO_2max and even greater during some practice sessions. In addition, this type of work is repeated daily, sometimes twice a day, six days a week for a large number of competitive swimmers.

One of the main reasons swimmers maintain this work ethic is that race requirements are supramaximal in nature. Thus, to elicit the metabolic and biomechanical factors required to perform at this intensity, it is common to train at supramaximal intensities to ensure optimal performance. However, a critical factor that is sometimes ignored is the intent of a specific swimming set. Specifically, the **actual** velocity and intensity that is maintained during a certain interval set. As the workout progresses, the amount of available carbohydrate will continually become depleted causing intensity/velocity to decrease. This is further complicated by the fact that most swim programs do not engage in fuel replenishment during practice and a majority of swimmers probably begin practice with an insufficient amount of glycogen. Ultimately, interval sets which are designed for a specific purpose are often not accomplished by the swimmer. Thus, a misadaptation in training occurs and the desired responses are not achieved.

An important component for fast swimming is achieving the highest possible work rate and being able to maintain at or near that work rate for a sustained period of time. However, if athletes continuously begin practice with low energy reserves and do not supplement during practice with high energy compounds, they will not be able to maintain critical swimming velocity during a specified training session. This, in effect will not induce severe stress to the glycolytic system and stimulate high-level energy turnover. Therefore, when the glycolytic system and high demand for rapid ATP production are challenged during competition, the swimmer is unable to respond to his/her full potential since practice sessions have failed to adequately train these systems.

5. References

1. Hermansen L. (1969) Anaerobic energy release. *Medicine and Science in Sport and Exercise* 1(1): 32-38.
2. Holloszy JO, Booth FW. (1976) Biochemical adaptations to endurance exercise in muscle. *Annual Physiological Reviews* 38: (273-291)
3. Holloszy JO, Coyle EF. (1984) Adaptations of skeletal muscle to endurance exercise and their metabolic consequenses. *Journal of Applied Physiology* 56: 831-838.
4. Morgan TE, Cobb LA, Short FA, Ross R, Gunn DL. (1971) Effect of long-term exercise on human muscle mitochondria. In: *Muscle Metabolism During Exercise.* (Pernow B & Saltin B, ed.) Plenum, New York, pp 87-95.
5. Costill DL, Flynn MG, Kirwan JP, Houmard JL, Mitchell JB, Fink WJ. (1988) Effects of repeated days of intensified training on muscle glycogen and swimming performance. *Medicine and Science in Sport and Exercise* 20: 249-254.
6. Saltin B, Rowell RB. (1980) Functional adaptations to physical activity and inactivity. *Federation Proceedings* 39: 1506-1513.
7. Gollnick PD, Armstrong RB, Saltin B, Saubert CW, Sembrowich WL, Shepherd RE. (1973) Effect of training on enzyme acitivity and fiber composition of human skeletal muscle. *Jouranl of Applied Physiology* 34(1): 107-111.
8. Lavoie J-M, Taylor AW, Montpetit RR. (1980) Skeletal muscle fibre size adaptation to an eight-week swimming programme. *Eurpoean Journal of Applied Physiology* 44: 161-165.
9. MacDougall JD, Elder GCB, Sale DG, Moroz JR, Sutton JR. (1980) Effects of strength training and immobilization on human muscle fibers. *Eurpoean Journal of Applied Physiology* 43: 25-34.
10. Fitts RH, Costill DL, Gardetto PR. (1989) Effect of swim exercise training on human muscle fiber function. *Journal of Applied Physiology* 66(1): 465-475.
11. Trappe SW. Anaerobic contributions: physiological and biochemical perspectives of elite sprint and endurance trained athletes [Thesis]. University of Colorado, 1991.
12. Krough A, Lindhard J. (1920) The changesin respiration at the transition from work to rest. *Journal of Physiology (London)* 53: 431-439.
13. Medbo JI, Mohn A-C, Tabata I, Bahr R, Vaage O, Sejersted OM. (1988) Anaerobic capacity determined by maximal accumulated O2 deficit. *Journal of Applied Physiology* 64(1): 50-60.
14. Medbo JI, Tabata I. (1989) Relative importance of aerobic and anaerobic energy release during short-lasting exhausting bicycle exercise. *Journal of Applied Physiology* 67(5): 1881-1886.
15. Medbo JI, Tabata I. (1993) Anaerobic energy release in working muscle during 30 s to 3 min of exhausting bicycling. *Journal of Applied Physiology* 75(4): 1654-1660.
16. Bergstrom J. (1962) Muscle electrolytes in man. *Scandinavian Journal of Clinical Laboratory Investigations* 14 (Suppl. 68): 7-110.
17. Passonneau JV, Lowry OH. (1993) *Enzymatic Analysis: A Practical Guide.* Humana Press, Inc., Totowa, NJ, pp 264-267.
18. Costill DL. (1992) Lactate metabolism for swimming. In: *Biomechanics and Medicine in Swimming: Swimming Science VI.* (Maclaren D, Reilly T, Lees A, ed.) E & FN Spon, London, pp. 3-11.
19. Fitts RH. (1994) Cellular mechanisms of muscle fatigue. *Physiological Reviews* 74(1): 49-94.
20. Bangsbo J, Gollnick PD, Graham TE, et al. (1990) Anaerobic energy production

and O2 deficit-debt relationship during exhaustive exercise in humans. *Journal of Physiology* 422(539-559.

21.   Saltin B. (1990) Anaerobic capacity: Past, present, and prospective. In: *Biochemistry of Exercise VII.* (Taylor AW, Gollnick PD, Green HJ, ed.) Human Kinetics, Champaign, IL, pp. 387-412.

19 DEVELOPING THE PREPUBERTAL ATHLETE: PHYSIOLOGICAL PRINCIPLES

O. BAR-OR
Children's Exercise & Nutrition Centre
McMaster University, Hamilton, Ontario, Canada

Abstract
There are several differences between the physiological responses of children and adults to exercise. To succeed in developing the child athlete, particularly in preparation for an athletic career that extends to adulthood, one must recognize these differences. This review focuses on the relationship between aerobic and anaerobic characteristics during growth, children's high metabolic cost of movement, faster recovery following exercise and deficient thermoregulatory capacity, as well on the trainability of their maximal aerobic power and muscle function. Practical recommendations, partially based on the above, are suggested.

1 Introduction

The successful preparation of children for an athletic career is comprised of several components. It starts with a proper selection of candidates, followed by a training regimen that must take into account the child's health and well-being (short- and long-term), unique physiological responses to exercise and to training, specific nutritional requirements associated with growth, and a variety of psychosocial considerations. Unlike with adult athletes, the team that prepares the child athlete must include the parents.

This article will highlight children's unique physiological responses to acute exercise and to training, and the practical implications thereof. When available, examples will be given regarding age-group swimmers. "Children" in this article denotes prepubescents. To review the psychosocial aspects of developing the young athlete see Gould [1], Weiss [2], Coakley [3] and Donnelly [4]. Principles of talent selection are described by Matsudo [5].

2 Uniqueness of Children's Physiological Responses to Exercise

2.1 Quantitative and Qualitative Age-Related Differences
Some differences in the exercise performance of children, adolescents and adults reflect qualitative morphological and functional differences. Others result from qualitative differences. For example, muscle strength is dependent upon its size. When calculated per cross-sectional area of the muscle, strength is similar in children, adolescents and young adults [6]. Likewise, maximal aerobic power, when expressed per kg body mass, lean leg mass or total blood

hemoglobin, is similar across these maturational groups [7]. In contrast, peak muscle power and local muscle endurance -- both reflecting "anaerobic" muscle characteristics -- are lower in children, even when corrected for body mass [8] or lean limb mass [9]. Indeed, longitudinal observations that measure both aerobic and anaerobic performance of boys reveal a growing ratio of anaerobic-to-aerobic peak power during puberty [10]. Likewise, the ratio of anaerobic-to-aerobic muscle enzyme activity is lower in children than in adolescents or young adults [11].

One implication of the above is that, compared with adults, children's athletic performance is particularly deficient in tasks such as jumping and sprint running and less deficient in endurance events. While this is true for track & field, it may not be so in swimming, where the percentage difference in performance between age-group and adult high-performance swimmers is similar in sprints and in long distances [12].

2.2 Metabolic Cost of Movement

When walking or running at a given speed, children have a higher oxygen uptake (VO_2) per kg body mass, compared with adolscents, who have a higher VO_2 than adults. Thus, the "metabolic reserve" (i.e., the difference between maximal VO_2 and that required for a submaximal task) is lowest in children [13]. This may be a major reason for the lower distance-running (and, possibly, swimming) performance of children, even when they compete against adults with a similar maximal VO_2. The causes for children's higher metabolic cost of locomotion are not clear, but preliminary kinematic and EMG data from the author's laboaratory suggest that the mechanical cost of locomotion is higher in children, as is the degree of co-contraction of their agonist and antagonist muscles groups. The latter causes a "waste" in metabolic demands.

2.3 Recovery Following Exercise

One physiological difference that gives children an advantage, is their faster recovery following aerobic [14] or anaerobic [15] exercise. After completing the Wingate anaerobic 30-s cycling test, boys could repeat the same mechanical power within 2 minutes, whereas young men required 10 min for their recovery [15]. A possible implication of this pattern is that children may need shorter rest periods during interval training than do adults.

2.4 Temperature Regulation and Dehydration

There are several morphological and physiological characteristics that make children less tolerant of prolonged exercise in extreme climatic heat or cold, compared with adults [16]. In 20-21C, for example, child swimmers have a much shorter tolerance time, compared with adolescent swimmers. For a given level of dehydration, children's core temperature rises faster than in adults. This may have health implications for child athletes who deliberately dehydrate, as in wrestling, or who incur "voluntary dehydration", as in distance running.

3 Uniqueness of Children's Trainability

"Trainability" denotes the extent of morphological and functional changes that are induced by training. In general, children respond to training in a similar manner to that of adults, but there are several quantitative differences in such responses.

3.1 Trainability of Maximal Aerobic Power

Obviously, aerobic training can improve children's performance (e.g., in swimming middle- and long distances). However, studies mostly from the 1970s and 1980s, have suggested that the aerobic system in prepubescents is either untrainable or less trainable than in more mature groups [17]. More recent studies show that, by undergoing training regimens similar to those practised by adult athletes, prepubescents are trainable [18]. To pass a definitive verdict regarding children's aerobic trainability, there is a need for studies across maturational groups, who are given an identical training stimulus.

3.2 Effects of Training on the Economy of Movement

Children who train for "aerobic" sports do not always have a higher maximal VO_2 than non-athletes. A case in point is a recent study which found little or no difference between the maximal VO_2 of prepubertal swimmers and non-athletes [19]. This seeming paradox may by reconciled by a training-induced increase in movement economy, unaccompanied by a higher maximal VO_2. This pattern has been found in young cross-country runners who, over several training seasons, kept decreasing their O_2 cost of running, without any increase in maximal VO_2 [20].

3.3 Effect of Training on Muscle Strength, Muscle Endurance and Peak Power

In spite of traditional beliefs that children cannot inncrease their muscle strength, there is now conclusive evidence that prepubertal girls and boys do respond to resistance training by an increase in their muscle strength [21]. The extent of such an increase, expressed as a percentage of pretraining strength, seems similar across maturational groups. One difference is that prepubescents can increase their strength without an increase in muscle bulk. One mechanism underlying this patttern is an increase in motor-unit activation, but there are possibly other neurological adaptations.

Likewise, training can increase a child's peak muscle power. This increase, however, is only 3-10%. The training-induced increase in local muscle endurance is apparently higher. There are no data comparing the trainability of these anaerobic charcteristics across maturational groups.

Whether an increase in muscle strength *per se* is accompanied by an improvement in children's sports performance is debatable. For example, supplementing a 6-week program by resistance training did not improve swim times of age-group swimmers [22]. In contrast, a more intensive and prolonged addition of resistance training did yield improved sprint-swimming times [23].

4 Practical Implications and Recommendations

The following are practical implications and recommendations regarding the development of the prepubertal athlete.

- It is seldom that a child's physical suitability for a specific event is established before puberty. Therefore, **a training regimen for a child athlete should be as varied as possible**, rather than focus on specialized tasks. Sports in which skill acquisition is the predominant component (e.g., gymnastics or figure skating) are an exception.

- Along the same line, there is **no proof that specialized training in children will yield long-range benefits**. For example, it is not clear whether a child who undergoes strength training before puberty will become a stronger adult.

- Before puberty, girls and boys have similar morphological and physiological characteristics. There is therefore **no physiological or medical reason why prepubescent girls and boys should not compete against each other,** even in contact and collision sports.

- Resistance training, using equipment modified for children and under adult supervision, is safe for prepubescents of both genders. There is no information, however, about the safety of competitve weight lifting or power lifting.

- Children take longer than adults to acclimatize to a warm environment. Therefore, upon transition from cool to warm climatic conditions, children should be given lighter training sessions for the first 10-14 days.

- Because children underestimate their fluid needs when exercising in warm environments, they should be encouraged to drink above and beyond their perceived thirst. To increase drinking volumes the child should be offered a flavored drink. Grape seems to be the flavor of choice for most children. Addition of salt and carbohydrates to the drink further enhances voluntary drinking volume.

5 References

1. Gould, D. (1993) Intensive sport participation and the prepubescent athlete: competitive stress and burnout, in *Intensive Participation in Children's Sports*, (eds. B.R. Cahill and A.J. Pearl), Human Kinetics, Champaign IL, pp. 19-38.
2. Weiss, M.R. (1993) Psychological effects of intensive sport participation on children and youth: self-esteem and motivation, in *Intensive Participation in Children's Sports*, (eds. B.R. Cahill and A.J. Pearl), Human Kinetics, Champaign IL, pp. 39-69.
3. Coakley, J. (1993) Social dimensions of intensive training and participation in youth sports, in *Intensive Participation in Children's Sports*, (eds. B.R. Cahill and A.J. Pearl), Human Kinetics, Champaign IL, pp. 77-94.
4. Donnelly, P. (1993) Problems associated with youth involvement in high-performance sport, in *Intensive Participation in Children's Sports*, (eds. B.R. Cahill and A.J. Pearl), Human Kinetics, Champaign IL, pp. 95-126.
5. Matsudo, V. (in press, 1995) Prediction of future athletic excellence, in *The Encyclopedia of Sports Medicine, Volume VI: The child and Adolescent Athlete* (Ed. O. Bar-Or), Benchmark Scientific Publications, London.
6. Davies, C.T.M. (1985) Strength and mechanical properties of muscle in children and young adults. *Scandinavian Journal of Sports Sciences*, Vol. 7, No. 5, pp. 11-5.
7. Astrand, P.-O. (1952) *Experimental Studies of Physical Working Capacity in Relation to Sex and Age*, Munksgaard, Copenhagen, pp. 1-171.
8. Inbar, O. and Bar-Or, O. (1986) Anaerobic characteristics in male children and adolescents. *Medicine and Science in Sports and Exercise*, Vol. 18, pp. 264-9.
9. Blimkie, C.J.R., Roche, P., Hay, J.T., and Bar-Or, O.. Anaerobic power of arms in

teenage boys and girls: relationship to lean tissue. *European Journal of Applied Physiology*, **Vol.** 57, pp. 677-83.

10. Falk, B. and Bar-Or, O. (1993) Longitudinal changes in peak aerobic and anaerobic mechanical power of circumpubertal boys. *Pediatric Exercise Science*, Vol. 5, pp. 318-31.

11. Berg, A. and Keul, J. (1988) Biochemical changes during exercise in children, in *Young Athletes: Biological, Psychological and Educational Perspectives*. (Ed. R.M. Malina), Human Kinetics, Champaign, IL, pp. 61-77.

12. Bar-Or, O., Unnithan, V., and Illecas, C. (in press, 1995) Physiologic considerations in age-group swimming. *Medicine and Sports Science*.

13. Bar-Or, O. (1983) *Pediatric Sports Medicine for the Practitioner: From Physiologic Principles to Clinical Applications*, Springer Verlag, New York.

14. Zanconato, S., Cooper, D.M., and Armon, Y. (1991) Oxygen cost and oxygen uptake dynamics and recovery with 1 min of exercise in children and adults. *Journal of Applied Physiology* Vol. 71, pp. 993-8.

15. Hebestreit, H., Mimura, K. and Bar-Or, O. (1993). Recovery of muscle power after high intensity short-term exercise: comparing boys and men. *Journal of Applied Physiology*, Vol. 74, pp. 2875-80.

16. Bar-Or, O. (1989) Temperature regulation during exercise in children and adolescents, in **Perspectives in Exercise and Sport Medicine Vol II**, (Eds. C. Gisolfi, and D.R. Lamb) Benchmark Press, ??? pp. 335-67.

17. Bar-Or, O. (1989) Trainability of the prepubescent child. *Physician and Sportsmedicine*, Vol. 17, No. 5, pp. 65-6; 75-82.

18. T.W. Rowland (1993) The Physiological impact of intensive training on the prepubertal athlete, in *Intensive Participation in Children's Sports*, (eds. B.R. Cahill and A.J. Pearl), Human Kinetics, Champaign IL, pp. 167-93.

19. Falgairette, P., Duche, P., Bedu N., Fellmann, N., and Coudert, J. (1993) Bioenergetic characteristics in prepubertal swimmers. *International Journal of Sports medicine*, Vol. 14, pp. 444-8.

20. Daniels, J., and Oldridge, N. (1971) Changes in oxygen consumption of young boys during growth and running training. *Medicine and Science in Sports*, Vol. 3, pp. 161-5.

21 Blimkie, C.J.R., and Bar-Or, O. (in press, 1995) Trainability of muscle Strength and power during childhood, in *The Encyclopedia of Sports Medicine, Volume VI: The child and Adolescent Athlete* (Ed. O. Bar-Or), Benchmark, London.

22. Ainsworth, J.L. (1970). *The effect of isometric-resistive exercises with the Exer-Genie on strength and speed in swimming*. Doctoral dissertation, University of Oklahoma.

23. Blanksby, B., and Gregor, J. (1981). Anthropometric, strength and physiological changes in male and female swimmers with progressive resistance training. *Australian Journal of Sport Sciences*, Vol. 1, 3-6.

20 ENERGY RELEASE DURING ALTITUDE AND ACUTE SIMULATED SEA LEVEL EXPOSURE IN ALTITUDE ACCLIMATIZED/TRAINED SWIMMERS

L.J. D'ACQUISTO*, Z.V. TRAN**, C.G.R. JACKSON** and J.P. TROUP***

*Central Washington University, Ellensburg, Washington USA
**University of Northern Colorado, Greeley, Colorado USA
***U.S. Swimming, University of Colorado, Colorado Springs, USA.

Abstract

Aerobic (Aer) and anaerobic (Anae) energy release were measured while swimming at altitude (A) (2000m, Pb=592mmHg) and in acute simulated sea level (ASSL) exposure (Pb=760mmHg) in moderate altitude acclimatized males. Subjects (n=10, 16.7+1.2 yr) resided (10.5+6.3yr) and swim trained (5.9+2.9yr) at altitude (2000m). An environmental chamber housing a swimming treadmill was used for all testing. Five submax (~20 to 70 %VO2 peak) and a max swim for determination of VO2 peak was performed. Anaerobic energy release for a max swim (100%VO2 peak) was derived by calculating the accumulated O2 deficit (AOD). A and ASSL VO2 peak was 3.70+0.11 (SE) and 4.17+0.13 l.min-1, (p<0.05). RPEmax, peak BLa (mM) and peak AOD at A and ASSL did not differ, (AOD, 4.32+0.33 vs 4.15+0.58 lO2 Eq). HRmax was lower during A (179.3+2.3bpm) vs ASSL (187.0+2.8bpm) (p<0.05). Saturation of hemoglobin with oxygen (SaO2) was 5% greater at ASSL vs A immediately following the VO2 peak swim (p<0.05). Percent relative VO2 peak, BLa and RPE submax were lower during ASSL (p<0.05). In summary: 1) peak aerobic energy delivery was increased in ASSL due to increased oxygen availability to the working musculature (enhanced SaO2 and HRmaX); 2) peak anaerobic energy release was independent of environmental condition; and 3) relative metabolic demand for submax swimming was lower in ASSL, suggesting faster swimming at a given percent of VO2 peak during acute sea level exposure in altitude acclimatized, trained swimmers.

Keywords: aerobic, altitude, anaerobic, oxygen deficit, swimming.

1 Introduction

Studies have illustrated that there are dramatic changes in metabolic responses during both maximal and submaximal exercise in sea level residents, who are well-trained, upon ascension to altitude [1,2,3,4]. At altitude the oxygen availability to the muscle cell is reduced, and consequently, maximal aerobic power is compromised [5]. A lowered maximal aerobic power results in reduced racing speeds, especially for more endurance oriented swimming events. An individuals ability to deliver energy anaerobically, however, is independent of altitude [5,6]. Therefore, swimming events which require a high anaerobic energy release (sprint events) are not compromised upon ascending to altitude conditions.

There are few studies which have examined the effects of an acute sea level exposure in well trained athletes who are long term residents of moderate altitude [7]. This is surprising, especially since so many athletes live and train at altitude for years and periodically travel to sea-level to compete. In view of the above, the purpose of this investigation was to examine the aerobic and anaerobic energy release at altitude and in acute simulated sea level conditions in moderate altitude (2000 m) acclimatized, trained swimmers.

2 Methods

2.1 Experimental design

Trained male swimmers (n=10) participated in this study after being informed of the possible risks and benefits associated with the project. Subjects had lived and swim trained at moderate altitude (1800-2000 meters) an average of 10.5 and 6.0 years, respectively. Subject characteristics (mean+SD) were as follows: age (yr), 16.7+1.2; height (cm), 175.5+10.7; weight (kg), 68.4+7.9; and, percent adipose tissue, 9.3+2.0.

Swimmers were tested at moderate altitude (2000 m; barometric pressure (Pb), 592mmHg) and during an acute (w/i three hours) simulated exposure to sea level (Pb=760mmHg). A swimming treadmill (flume) housed in an environmental chamber was used for all testing. Measurements were first completed at altitude followed one week later with testing at simulated sea level conditions. Subjects were familiar with all testing procedures.

2.2 Testing procedure

Metabolic. The first testing session consisted of subjects completing a swimming economy profile which consisted of five, six minute submaximal (~20 to 70%VO2 peak; 0.9 to 1.3 m.s-1) swims. VO2 values collected during the final two minutes were averaged to determine steady state VO2. An incremental maximal swim to volitional exhaustion for to determine VO2 peak was performed twenty minutes following the last submaximal swim bout. Heart rate was monitored manually by the same technician immediately following each swim effort. Rating of perceived exertion was also assessed immediately following the submaximal and VO2 peak swims [8].

In a second session, swimmers performed a maximal swim (100%VO2 peak) to volitional exhaustion. Peak anaerobic energy release was assessed by calculating the accumulated oxygen deficit (AOD) [9]. AOD is equal to the total oxygen demand (TOD) minus the accumulated oxygen uptake (AOU) of the maximal swim [9].

Biochemistry. A finger stick immediately following each submaximal swim effort and 1, 3, 5, 7, and 9 minutes post maximal swim was performed to determine steady state and peak blood lactate (mM) levels, respectively (YSI blood lactate analyzer). In addition, a sample of blood taken immediately post max swim was analyzed for saturation of hemoglobin with oxygen (SaO2) (Instrumentation Labs-1312 Blood-Gas Analyzer).

Statistics. Means, standard deviations and standard errors were computed. A two-way analysis of variance with repeated measures (SPSS) was used to analyze the data. A Tukey post hoc test was used when a significant overall F value was found. Level of significance was set a priori at the 0.05 level.

3 Results

3.1 Metabolic
Peak VO2 (l.min-1) during ASSL exposure, 4.17+0.13 (SE), was significantly greater than during moderate altitude testing, 3.70+0.11 (Figure 1). Heart rate max was greater during ASSL exposure (187+2.8bpm) when compared to moderate altitude (179.3+2.3bpm)($p < 0.05$).

The percent difference in VO2 between altitude and an ASSL exposure at 0.9, 1.0, 1.1, 1.2, and 1.3 m.s-1 was 26.2, 15.1, 14.9, 7.65, and 4.65, respectively ($p < 0.05$). Relative swimming intensity (percent of VO2 peak) was significantly reduced for all submaximal swimming efforts during ASSL. RPE was significantly lower for all submaximal efforts during ASSL; however, no difference was found for RPE following the maximal VO2 peak swim. Peak accumulated oxygen deficit for ASSL and Altitude was 4.15+0.58 and 4.32+0.33 l O2 Eq., respectively ($p > 0.05$) (Figure 1).

3.2 Biochemistry
Peak blood lactate at altitude and ASSL was 10.65+0.72 mM and 9.16+0.28 mM, respectively ($p > 0.05$). Blood lactate levels at 0.9, 1.0, 1.1, 1.2, and 1.3 m.s-1 were 35, 15, 22, 40 and 6 percent lower during the ASSL submaximal swims, respectively ($p < 0.05$). SaO2 immediately following the maximal swim (VO2 peak test) was significantly lower at altitude (91.39+0.76%) when compared to sea level (96.27+0.24%).

4 Discussion

An eleven percent increase in peak aerobic power with an increase in barometric pressure (592 to 760mmHg) explains, in part, why endurance oriented performances are enhanced when altitude acclimatized, trained swimmers compete at sea level. The difference of 11% in peak aerobic power is in agreement with a recent investigation examining the effect of a hypobaric hypoxic environment on seven trained male collegiate swimmers who resided at sea level [10]. In the latter study by Ogita and Tabata (1992) a 12% difference in VO2 peak (4.15+0.18 vs 3.65+0.11 l.min-1) was found between sea level and a simulated altitude of 2000 meters. It should be noted that the average VO2 peak values reported by Ogita and Tabata (1992) are very similar to values reported in the present investigation, 4.17+0.13 l.min-1 at simulated sea level and 3.70+ l.min-1 during altitude testing.

In comparing the findings of the present investigation with Ogita and Tabata's study (1992) of trained swimmers (sea level residents) tested at sea level and during hypobaric hypoxia, it is tempting to speculate that perhaps long term swim training (years) at moderate altitude does not enhance sea level peak VO2. This speculation is based on the fact that the average sea level VO2 peak value (3.65+0.11 l.min-1) for the sea level trained swimmers in the Ogita and Tabata study was not different than the the average VO2 peak value measured during hyperbaric normoxia for moderate altitude acclimatized (2000 meters) swimmers in the present study (3.70+0.11 l.min-1).

Further support for the above speculation was presented in a study by Grover and Reeves [7]. This study compared various metabolic parameters of athletes residing at near sea level (330m) with athletes native to medium altitude (3100m). The athletes native to altitude had a history of participating in either skiing, basketball, or American football. The sea level athletes were active in track. When the sea level residents were tested at altitude, VO2 max on the day of arrival decreased 25%. Altitude residents had a 27% increase in VO2 max when tested at sea level. These investigators concluded that living at moderate altitude does not reduce the handicap on the oxygen transport system during maximal exercise at altitude. Furthermore, living and training at altitude did not provide an added advantage in maximal aerobic power during sea level testing. In other words, VO2 max at sea level for the altitude residents was similar to that of the sea level residents.

The increased VO2 peak at sea level can be explained by an enhanced oxygen availability to the working muscles. The latter is justified by the greater saturation of hemoglobin with oxygen (SaO2)(91.4% vs 96.3%) at sea level conditions and also a higher heart rate max (179 bpm vs 187 bpm). The increased SaO2 can be explained by a greater barometric pressure at sea level and consequently an increased driving pressure for oxygen to diffuse from the alveoli into the pulmonary blood. The lowered heart rate max at altitude is in disagreement with previous experimental findings [1,7] but in agreement with those by Daniels (personal communication, November 1992) and several other investigators [4,11]. Daniels, for example, found an average decrease of 10 bpm for maximal heart rate in distance runners at an altitude of 2250 meters. There is no clear explanation as to the descrepancies found in the literature on heart rate max between sea level and altitude conditions.

This investigation suggests that altitude acclimatized trained swimmers become more economical when swimming under normoxic conditions. Previous studies have illustrated no change [10 (swimmers)] or a decrease [1 (distance runners)] in oxygen consumption during submaximal exercise between altitude (2000-2300 meters) and sea level conditions. The increased VO2 peak coupled with improved swimming economy under sea level conditions resulted in a reduction in the relative metabolic demand for submax swimming. This suggests faster swimming at a given percent of VO2 peak during sea level exposure in altitude acclimatized, trained swimmers.

The general comment made by subjects while swimming under simulated sea level conditions was that it "felt easier". This was reflected by a reduced rating of perceived exertion for all submax efforts. Percent effort as related to VO2 peak was reduced during the submaximal sea level swimming bouts, suggesting that the relative swimming intensity is a critical determinant of perceived exertion. In addition, blood lactate level was lower during the submaximal swim bouts at sea level, providing further evidence of a reduced submaximal metabolic load.

Despite a significant increase in peak VO2 during the simulated sea level exposure, anaerobic energy release remained unaffected (Figure 1). This finding clearly illustrates that peak anaerobic energy delivery is independent of peak aerobic energy production. The latter finding makes it clear that swimming events which are sprint oriented will be minimally affected by descending to sea level while endurance events will experience the most improvement.

5 References

1. Squires, R.W. and Buskirk, E.R.(1982) Aerobic capacity during acute exposure to simulated altitude, 914 to 2286 meters. *Medicine and Science in Sports and Exercise*, Vol. 14, No. 1. pp.36-40.

2. D'Acquisto, L.J., Trappe, S.W., Franciosi, P., Takahashi, S., and Troup, J.P.(1991) *Effects of acute altitude exposure on the aerobic:anaerobic demands of swimming.* Medicine and Science in Sports and Exercise, Vol. 23, No. 4. (Suppl.), p. S91.

3. Buskirk, E., Kollias, J., Akers, R., Prokop, E., and Reatequi, E.(1967) Maximal performance at altitude and on return from altitude in conditioned runners. *Journal of Applied Physiology*, Vol. 23, pp. 259-266.

4. Faulker, J., Kollias, J., Favour, C., Guskirk, E., and Balke, B.(1968) Maximal aerobic capacity and running performance at altitude. *Journal of Applied Physiology*, Vol. 24, pp. 685-691.

5. Astrand, P. and Rodahl, K.(1986) *Textbook of Work Physiology* (3rd ed.). McGraw-Hill Publisher, New York.

6. Linnarsson, D., Karlsson, J., Fagraeus, Saltin, B. (1974) Muscle metabolites and oxygen deficit with exercise in hypoxia and hyperoxia. *Journal of Applied Physiology*, Vol. 36, No.4, pp. 399-402.

7. Grover, R.F. and Reeves, J.T.(1967) Exercise performance of athletes at sea level and 3100 meters altitude. In. R.F. Goodard(Ed.), *The effects of altitude on physical performance*, The Athletic Institute, Chicago. pp. 80-87.

8. Borg, G.(1970) Perceived exertion as an indicator of somatic stress. *Scandinavian Journal of Rehabilitative Medicine*, Vol. 2, pp. 92-98.

9. Medbo, J.L., Mohn, A.C., Tabata, I., Bahr, R., Vaage, O., and Sejersted, O.M.(1988) Anaerobic capacity determined by maximal O2 deficit. *Journal of Applied Physiology*, Vol. 64, No. 1, pp. 50-60.

10. Ogita, F. and Tabata, I.(1992) Oxygen uptake during swimming in a hypobaric environment. *European Journal of Applied Physiology*, Vol. 65, pp. 192-196.

11. Dill, D.B. and Adams, W.(1971) Maximal oxygen uptake at sea level and 3,090m in high school champion runners. *Journal of Applied Physiology*, Vol. 30, pp. 854-859.

21 DETERMINATION AND VALIDITY OF CRITICAL SWIMMING FORCE AS PERFORMANCE INDEX IN TETHERED SWIMMING

Y. IKUTA
Department of Physical Education, Osaka University of Education, Kashiwara, Japan

K. WAKAYOSHI
Laboratory of Health & Sports Science, Nara University of Education, Nara, Japan

T. NOMURA
Institute of Health and Sports Sciences, University of Tsukuba, Japan

Abstract
The purpose of this investigation was to determine whether the concepts of critical swimming velocity (v_{cri}) and critical power (w_{cri}) could be applied in tethered swimming as critical swimming force (f_{cri}), and whether f_{cri} could be utilized as an effective index for assessing endurance performance in competitive swimmers. The subjects who volunteered for this study were thirteen male trained collegiate swimmers (18-21 years). The subjects were instructed to swim four times in tethered swimming.

The regression equations between impulse (i) and maximal sustained time (t) were expressed in the general form, $i=a+b*t$, with r value being higher than 0.996 ($p<0.01$). Furthermore, v_{cri}, swimming velocity corresponding 4 mmol*l^{-1} of blood lactate concentration (v_{OBLA}) and mean velocity in the 400 m free style maximal effort (v_{400}) were measured on each subject. Significant correlations were found between f_{cri} and v_{400} ($r=0.703$, $p<0.01$), f_{cri} and v_{cri} ($r=0.691$, $p<0.01$), and f_{cri} and v_{OBLA} ($r=0.682$, $p<0.05$). These data suggested that f_{cri} could be defined as the force of tethered swimming which could be theoretically maintained without exhaustion and could be adopted as an index for assessing endurance performance.
Keywords: Competitive swimming, Critical swimming force, Critical swimming velocity, Tethered swimming.

1 Introduction

The concept of the critical power (w_{cri}) found by Monod and Scherrer [1] was expanded by many studies [2] [3] [4]. Recently, Wakayoshi et al. [5] [6] [7] had applied to the field of swimming, and found a new concept of the critical swimming velocity (v_{cri}). v_{cri}, defined as the swimming velocity which could be theoretically maintained forever without exhaustion, was expressed as the slope of the regression line between swimming distance and its duration. Moreover, Wakayoshi et al. [8] indicated that v_{cri} corresponded to the swimming velocity at maximal lactate steady state level and could be adopted as an index of endurance ability.

The purpose of this investigation was to determine whether the concepts of v_{cri} and w_{cri} could be applied as critical swimming force (f_{cri}) which could theoretically be maintained without exhaustion during tethered swimming, and whether f_{cri} could be utilized as an effective index for assessing endurance performance in competitive swimmers.

2 Methods

2.1 Subjects
The subjects who volunteered for this study were thirteen male trained collegiate swimmers (18-21 years).

2.2 Determination of v_{cri}
The v_{cri} was determined by a two-trial test [8]. In this test, the subjects were instructed to swim the distance of 200 and 400 m at maximal effort in the long course swimming pool. By plotting each subject's swimming distance against duration time and connecting two data points, v_{cri} could be determined by the slope of the line. The test was carried out 1 event per day.

2.3 Determination of v_{OBLA}
The swimming velocity corresponding 4 mmol$*$l^{-1} of blood lactate concentration (v_{OBLA}) was determined by two-speed test of Olbrecht et al. [9]. The subjects swam 400 m twice: once at a constant velocity of 85% of their best time of 400 m free style and once at maximal effort . A resting period of more than 40 min was allowed between two trials. Capillary blood was taken from the finger tip before and 3 min after each trial. Blood lactate was analyzed by an enzymatic membrane method (YSI23L, Yellow Springs Instruments), which had been calibrated using a standard concentration of lactate. By plotting each subject's blood lactate concentrations against swimming velocity and connecting two data points, v_{OBLA} could be determined by interpolation or extrapolation.

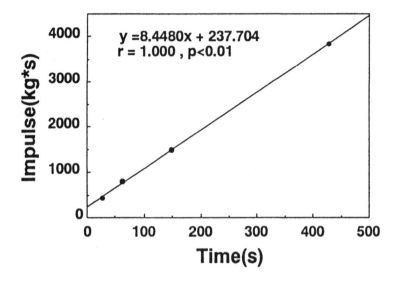

Fig. 1.   Relationship between the impulse and the maximal sustainable time plotted from the data of subject 1.

2.4 Determination of f_{cri}

The subjects were instructed to swim four times in the tethered swimming. When a subject swims at a steady load in the tethered swimming, exercise usually ceases at a fairly well-defined point, i.e. the subject can no longer keep up the predetermined load.

The steady-state loads employed in the tethered swimming were four constant forces ranging from 6.5 to 16.0 kg. The lowest tethered force was set as the exercise intensity at which each subject could continue to swim longer than 4 min. Rest periods of at least 30 min between the test periods were allowed.

Fig. 1 illustrates the determination of f_{cri} based upon the concept of w_{cri} [1] and v_{cri} [5] [6] [7] [8]. In the present study, f_{cri} has been defined as the tethered force which could theoretically be maintained without fatigue. The impulse obtained from four constant forces were plotted as a function of the maximal time. These points were accurately situated on a line defined by the relationship between impulse (i) and maximal sustainable time (t). Tethered force (f) multiplied by t makes i:

$$i = f * t \qquad\qquad (1)$$

The equation of the regression line can be expressed as follows :

$$i = a + b * t \tag{2}$$

i can be substituted by $f * t$ from equation 1, giving:

$$f * t = a + b * t \tag{3}$$
$$f = a * t^{-1} + b \tag{4}$$

Theoretically, if we could set the tethered force at a level which could be performed indefinitely ($t \varnothing$_), $a*t^{-1}$ would approach zero and f would approach b.

Therefore, f_{cri} can be expressed as the slope of the regression line :

$$f_{cri} = b \tag{5}$$

3 Results

Table 1 shows the subjects' physical characteristics, the speciality swimming styles, and the data obtained from the tests in the present study. Velocity of the 400 m free style (v_{400}) ranged from 1.274 to 1.516 $m*s^{-1}$, with a mean of 1.425 $m*s^{-1}$ (SD=0.075). It is apparent that the subjects in the present study are relatively homogeneous with regard to their performance (v_{400}) having coefficients of variation of 5.3%. v_{cri} calculated by the two-trial test ranged from 1.171 to 1.400 $m*s^{-1}$ with a mean of 1.327 $m*s^{-1}$ (SD=0.066). v_{OBLA} calculated by the two-speed test ranged from 1.211 to 1.417 $m*s^{-1}$ with a mean of 1.313 $m*s^{-1}$ (SD=0.073).

Table 1. Physical characteristics and test results for each subject

Subject	Height (cm)	Mass (kg)	Age (year)	Speciality	v_{400} (m/s)	v_{cri} (m/s)	v_{OBLA} (m/s)	f_{cri} (kg)
1	178.0	76.0	19	FLY	1.470	1.377	1.321	8.448
2	178.0	74.0	20	FR-S	1.488	1.367	1.370	8.796
3	170.0	58.5	18	IM	1.467	1.334	1.357	7.098
4	181.0	71.0	21	FR-M	1.516	1.400	1.407	6.778
5	178.0	68.0	19	IM	1.477	1.368	1.370	7.095
6	182.5	65.0	20	FR-L	1.460	1.383	1.417	7.548
7	163.0	58.0	20	BA	1.373	1.280	1.236	5.813
8	180.0	80.0	20	FR-S	1.462	1.360	1.330	7.608
9	165.0	65.0	19	FR-M	1.394	1.300	1.280	6.144
10	170.0	73.0	20	FLY	1.314	1.271	1.223	6.200
11	169.0	63.0	20	FR-L	1.475	1.380	1.333	6.396
12	178.0	71.0	21	FR-S	1.350	1.264	1.219	5.637
13	175.0	68.0	20	IM	1.274	1.171	1.211	5.729
Mean	174.4	68.5	19.8		1.425	1.327	1.313	6.868
SD	6.317	6.564	0.832		0.075	0.066	0.073	1.019

Table 2. Correlation matrix for variables measured by each experiment

	v_{400}	v_{cri}	v_{OBLA}	f_{cri}
v_{400}	1			
v_{cri}	0.959**	1		
v_{OBLA}	0.914**	0.885**	1	
f_{cri}	0.703**	0.691**	0.682*	1

*p<0.05, **p<0.01

The experimental plots used to determine f_{cri} of subject 1 are shown in Fig. 1 as an example. The regression equation between i and t were expressed in the general form, i=a+b*t, with r value being higher than 0.996 (p<0.01). These results shown extremely good linearity. f_{cri} ranged from 5.637 to 8.796 kg with a mean of 6.868 kg (SD=1.019).

Results presented in Table 2 show the relationships between f_{cri}, v_{400}, v_{cri} and v_{OBLA}. Significant positive correlations were found between f_{cri} and v_{400} (r=0.703, p<0.01), f_{cri} and v_{cri} (r=0.691, p<0.01) and f_{cri} and v_{OBLA} (r=0.682, p<0.05). Furthermore, significant positive correlations were found between v_{OBLA} and v_{400} (r=0.914, p<0.01), v_{OBLA} and v_{cri} (r=0.885, p<0.01) and v_{cri} and v_{400} (r=0.959, p<0.01).

4 Discussion

One of the goal of this study was to calculate f_{cri}, and to confirm the possibility of application the concepts of v_{cri} and w_{cri} to the tethered swimming. Another was to assess the f_{cri} could be the index of endurance ability of competitive swimmers.

Since the tethered swimming has the function to keep a constant intensity similar to the swimming flume and the cycle ergometry, which were used the measuring the v_{cri} and w_{cri} in the previous studies [2] [3] [4] [6] [7], it is thought that it is possible to determine the f_{cri} by using the tethered swimming method.

In the present study, a strong correlation between i and t (r>0.996) was found for every subject, so that the relationship i=a+b*t was remarkably linear. Therefore, this result suggests that the concept of f_{cri} can be applied to competitive swimming and can be defined as the force of tethered swimming which can be theoretically maintained without exhaustion.

Many studies were reported that v_{400}, v_{OBLA} and v_{cri} were good indices as assessing the endurance ability [5] [6] [7] [8] [9]. In the present study, there are significant positive correlations between f_{cri} and endurance indices such as v_{400}, v_{OBLA} and v_{cri}. Therefore, it seems reasonable to suppose that f_{cri} can be adopted as an index for assessing the endurance ability. Furthermore, Wakayoshi et al. [8] reported that v_{cri}

may correspond to the exercise intensity at maximal lactate steady state. Consequently, it can not be denied that the f_{cri} determined the tethered swimming may correspond to the swimming intensity at maximal lactate steady state level.

5 References

1. Monod, H. and Scherrer, J. (1965) The work capacity of a synergic muscular group. *Ergonomics*, Vol. 8, pp. 329-37.
2. Moritani, T., Nagata, A., deVries,H.A. and Muro, M. (1981) Critical power as a measure of physical work capacity and anaerobic threshold. *Ergonomics*, Vol. 24, pp. 339-50.
3. deVries,H.A., Moritani, T., Nagata, A. and Magnussen, K. (1982) The relation between critical power and neuromuscular fatigue as estimated from electromyographic data. *Ergonomics*, Vol. 25, pp. 783-91.
4. Nagata, A., Moritani, T. and Muro, M. (1983) Critical power as a measure of muscular fatigue and anaerobic threshold. In: *Biomechanics VIIIA*, (ed. Matsui,H., Kobayashi, K.), Human Kinetics, Champaign, Ill., pp.312-20.
5. Wakayoshi, K., Yoshida, T., Kasai, T., Moritani, T., Mutoh, Y. and Miyashita, M. (1992) Validity of critical velocity as swimming fatigue threshold in the competitive swimmer. *Ann. Physiol. Anthrop.* Vol. 11, pp.301-7.
6. Wakayoshi, K., Ikuta, K., Yoshida, T., Udo, M., Moritani, T., Mutoh, Y. and Miyashita, M. (1992) Determination and validity of critical velocity as an index of swimming performance in the competitive swimmer. *Eur. J. Appl. Physiol.* Vol. 64, pp. 153-7.
7. Wakayoshi, K., Yoshida, T., Udo, M., Kasai, T., Moritani, T., Mutoh, Y. and Miyashita, M. (1992) A simple method for determining critical speed as swimming fatigue threshold in competitive swimming. *Int. J. Sports. Med.* Vol.13, pp. 367-71.
8. Wakayoshi, K., Yoshida, T., Udo, M., Harada, T., Moritani, T.,Mutoh, Y. and Miyashita, M. (1993) Does critical swimming velocity represent exercise intensity at maximal lactate steady state ?. *Eur. J. Appl. Physiol.* Vol. 66, pp. 90-5.
9. Olbrecht, J., Madsen, O., Mader, A., Liesen, H. and Hollmann, W. (1985) Relationship between swimming velocity and lactic concentration during continuous and intermittent training exercise. *Int. J. Sports. Med.* Vol.6, pp. 74-7.

22 RELATIONSHIP BETWEEN METABOLIC PARAMETERS AND STROKING TECHNIQUE CHARACTERISTICS IN FRONT CRAWL

K. WAKAYOSHI
Laboratory of Health & Sports Science, Nara University of Education, Nara, Japan

J. D'ACQUISTO
Exercise Science Laboratoty Central Washington University, Ellensburg, USA

J.M. CAPPAERT and J.P. TROUP
International Center for Aquatic Research, Colorado Springs, USA

Abstract

The purpose of this study was to determine the relationship between physiological parameters and stroking technique characteristics in front crawl. Subjects performed a swimming economy test for determination of steady-state oxygen uptake (VO2) and an incremental swim test to volitional exhaustion for determination of peak aerobic power (VO2peak). Two additional swim efforts were performed at velocities corresponding to 80 and 100%VO2peak (V80%VO2peak and V100%VO2peak). Stroke length (SL), stroke rate (SR) and velocity at the onset of blood lactate accumulation (VOBLA) were determined to assess stroking technique and endurance ability. For each sub-maximal effort, SL and SR remained unchanged throughout the six minute swim, and VO2 was found to reach steady-state levels. During the 80 and 100%VO2peak swims, SL and SR showed significant decreases and increases, respectively. VO2 increased significantly throughout the 80 and 100% VO2peak swims. Lactate threshold (LT) corresponded to an average velocity of 1.3 m/s and a mean VOBLA of 1.423±0.017 m/s. These results suggest that stroking technique remained unchanged during swimming activities corresponding to aerobic intensities, but changes in swimming mechanics occurred in order to maintain pace at anaerobic workloads.

Keywords: Oxygen uptake, blood lactate, stroke rate, stroke length

1 Introduction

Swimming velocity is the product of SR and SL and increases or decreases in velocity are due to a combined increase or decrease in SR and SL, respectively. Craig and Pendergast [1] reported that increases in velocity are predominantly produced by increases in SR, with smaller decreases in SL. Costill et al. [2] presented the concept of stroke index (SI), which is the product of swimming velocity and SL, and indicated that SI was the best predictor of VO2max in trained swimmers. Keskinen and Komi [3], and Weiss et al. [4], who studied the relationship between the changes of SR and SL and blood lactate concentrations (La), reported that an increase in SR and a decrease in SL became progressively greater when the intensity increased over the LT and OBLA. However, to date there have been no investigations examining the relationship between VO2 and stroking characteristics in intensities corresponding to both aerobic and anaerobic workloads.

Therefore, the purpose of this study was to determine the relationship between physiological parameters (VO2 and blood lactate) and stroking technique characteristics (SR and SL) at aerobic to anaerobic intensities.

2 Methods

2.1 Subjects and swimming flume
The subjects who volunteered for this study were eight trained male swimmers (16.9± 0.4 years, Mean±SE). All swimming tests were performed in a specially designed swimming flume in which velocity could be controlled from 0 to 3.0 m/s.

2.2 Measurement of VO2peak
VO2peak was measured by an incremental swim test to volitional exhaustion. Swimming velocity started at 1.3 m/s for the first two min followed by an increase of 0.05 m/s every half min until volitional exhaustion. During the incremental test, subjects breathed through a low resistance valve assembly. Expired gas was analyzed on-line every 10 s for measurements of VO2 and carbon dioxide output (VCO2). The two consecutive highest VO2 values during the incremental swim test were averaged and determined as VO2peak.

2.3 Swimming economy test
The swimming economy test [5] consisted of five (0.9, 1.0, 1.1, 1.2 and 1.3 m/s) sub-maximal swims. The subjects were instructed to swim for 6 min at each velocity with a four minute rest between each swim. To determine steady state oxygen uptake all sub-maximal efforts were performed at intensities ranging from approximately 30% to 60% VO2peak. During the swimming economy test, VO2, VCO2 and VE were determined by averaging metabolic values collected during the last 1 min of each sub-maximal swim.

The regression equation between VO2 and velocity cubed (V3) was represented by the following formula (Fig. 1).

$$VO2 = a + b*V3 \quad (1)$$

V80%VO2peak and V100%VO2peak were calculated by substituting the 80 and 100% VO2peak values into each subjects regression equation (1). Two additional six-min swim tests at V80%VO2peak and V100%VO2peak were performed. All subjects could not continue to swim at V100%VO2peak over the full 6 min.

2.4 Determination of onset of blood lactate accumulation (OBLA)
OBLA has previously been used for evaluating endurance ability [6]. By plotting La against velocity, it was possible to calculate VOBLA corresponding to 4 mM. Arterialized capillary blood was taken from the finger tip immediately after each sub-maximal swim, and 1, 3, 5, 7, and 9 min following the 100% VO2peak swim test.

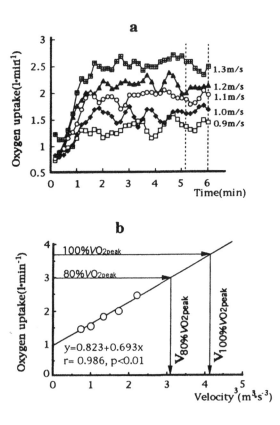

Fig. 1. Changes of VO2 on the swimming economy test (a) and a relationship between VO2 and velocity cubed (V3) (b)

Table 1. The physical characteristics and test results for each subjects

Subj.	Age (yrs)	VO2peak (l/min)	VO2peak/kg (ml/min/kg)	V80%VO2peak (m/s)	V100%VO2peak (m/s)	VOBLA (m/s)
MF	17	3.08	57.79	1.398	1.535	1.410
PT	18	4.16	58.23	1.632	1.790	1.489
DT	16	3.87	51.86	1.429	1.578	1.363
BL	15	3.69	47.99	1.460	1.618	1.381
MJ	16	3.21	55.07	1.490	1.643	1.367
GW	18	4.03	55.18	1.570	1.718	1.467
RO	17	4.13	58.18	1.696	1.866	1.465
TR	18	3.74	51.86	1.605	1.765	1.439
Mean	16.7	3.68	54.27	1.507	1.658	1.412
SE	0.4	0.13	1.05	0.036	0.038	0.017

2.5 Measurement of SR and SL

During the swimming economy test and six-min swim tests at V80%VO2peak and V100%VO2peak, five stroke cycles were timed during each 30 s block for all swims. SR (stroke/s) was calculated from the average value of the two measurements within each minute. SL (m/stroke) was calculated by dividing velocity by SR.

3 Results

VO2peak ranged from 3.08 to 4.16 (3.68±.13, Mean±SE) l/min. VOBLA ranged from 1.363 to 1.489 (1.412±.017) m/s is significantly lower than V80%VO2peak (1.398 to 1.696, 1.507±.036 m/s) and V100%VO2peak (1.535 to 1.866, 1.658±.038 m/s) (Table 1).

Fig. 1 illustrates an example (subject BL) for the result of the swimming economy test. Fig. 1a shows VO2 during various sub-maximal steady-state swimmings in relation to time and Fig. 1b indicates a relationship between average VO2 for last 1 min and velocity cubed. Correlation coefficients between VO2 and V3 ranged from 0.963 to 0.998 (p<0.01) and these regression equations were utilized to calculate V80%VO2peak and V100%VO2peak.

Fig. 2 shows the changes in averages of VO2, SR and SL for all subjects as a function of time at seven constant velocities from sub-maximal to maximal swims. At the sub-maximal effort swims (0.9 to 1.3 m/s), VO2 increased progressively to a steady-state level between 3 and 6 min, and SR and SL reached a steady-state from first to last minute. At V80%VO2peak and V100%VO2peak, however, VO2 was found to significantly increase throughout the tests, and SL and SR showed significant decrease and increase, respectively.

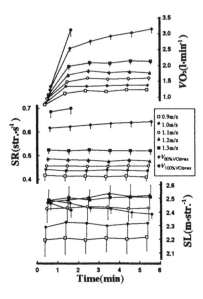

Fig. 2. Changes in averages of VO2, SR and SL for all subjects as a function of time at seven constant velocities.

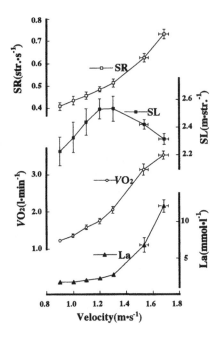

Fig. 3. Relationships between SR, SL, VO2, and La, and velocity at sub-maximal and maximal efforts.

Fig. 3 illustrates the relationships between SR, SL, VO2, and La, and velocity at sub-maximal and maximal efforts. SR, VO2 and La showed abrupt increases with velocity up to 1.3 m/s, whereas SL increased below 1.2 m/s and decreased above 1.3 m/s. The averages of VO2 for last 1 minute at 1.3 m/s, VOBLA, V80%VO2peak and V100%VO2peak corresponded to 57%, 72%, 85% and 96% of VO2peak, respectively.

4 Discussion

Previous studies have reported that the anaerobic threshold (AT) corresponds to an exercise intensity ranging from 60 to 70% VO2peak [7, 8]. The present study found that blood lactate levels ranged from 1 to 3 mM for swimming intensities below 60% VO2peak. In addition, swimming intensities at V80%VO2peak and V100%VO2peak resulted in average blood lactate levels of 6 and greater than 10 mM, respectively. The aforementioned studies [7, 8] and the blood lactate results suggest that swims performed at 30 to 60% VO2peak and those efforts swum at 85% and 96% VO2peak were below and above the AT, respectively. Consequently, it can also be established that the lower intensity efforts required a greater aerobic energy contribution relative to the higher velocities swims. While swimming at highly aerobic intensities it is clear that stroking technique remained constant throughout the entire six minute, steady state swim. In contrast, results of this study showed a significant increase in SR, a decrease in SL, and a progressive increase in VO2, during the more demanding swims (85% and 96% VO2peak). This inverse change in stroking mechanics during the latter part of the swims suggests a reduction in stroke technique since more strokes per given time were required to maintain the same pace. A reduction in stroke technique was most likely a result of the swimmer's inability to maintain a feel for the water, as noted by the reduced distance covered per stroke, which was perhaps attributable to local muscular fatigue.

Findings of an inverse change in stroking mechanics during more anaerobically demanding swims are consistent with previous results reported by craig [9] and Wakayoshi et al. [10] who have showed a tendency for SL to decrease during the latter stages of a competitive swim race. Keskinen and Komi [3] attributed a reduction in stroking mechanics (reduced SL) to muscle fatigue as the velocity increased over lactate threshold pace.

Most racing speeds in swimming require a high anaerobic power output, therefore it does not make sense to workout frequently and for prolong periods of time in low intensity training bouts. This study suggests that swimmers must work out at intensities which are specific to their racing speed. Practicing at racing speeds will mimic most closely the dynamics of stroking mechanics experienced during competition. Coaches should make an attempt to determine where stroke rate increases and stroke length decreases occur during a competitive race. It is at this biomechanical turning point that swimmers should practice at maintaining stroke length while increasing stroke rate.

In conclusion, it was found that 1)stroking technique remains unchanged during low intensity, steady state swimming (30 to 60% VO2peak), and 2) a biomechanical turning point (increased SR and reduced SL) occurs in the latter stages of swim bouts which are above the anaerobic threshold. In summary, it is important that the coaches prescribe workouts that allow the swimmer to experience the same stroking technique dynamics as in competition.

5 References

1. Craig, A.B. and Pendergast, D.R. (1979) Relationships of stroke rate, distance per stroke, and velocity in competitive swimming. *Med. Sci. Sports Exerc.*, Vol. 11, pp. 278-83.

2. Costill, D., Kovaleski, J., Porter, D., Kirwan, J., Fielding, R. and King, D. (1985) Energy expenditure during front crawl swimming: predicting success in middle-distance events. *Int. J. Sports Med.*, Vol. 6, pp. 266-70.

3. Keskinen, K.L. and Komi, P.V. (1993) Stroking characteristics of front crawl swimming during exercise. *J. Appl. Biomechanics*, Vol. 9, pp. 219-26.

4. Weiss, M., Reischle, K., Bouws, N., Simon, G. and Weicker, H. (1988) Relationship of blood lactate accumulation to stroke rate and distance per stroke in top female swimmers. *Swimming science V*, (ed. B.E. Ungerechts, K. Wilke and K. Reischle), Champaign, IL, pp. 295-303.

5. D'Acquisto, L.J., Barzdukas, A.P., Dursthoff, P., Letner, C. and Troup, J.P. (1992) Physiological adaptations to 60 vs 20 minutes of swim training at 76% VO2max. Biomechanics and medicine in swimming, *Swimming Science VI*, (ed. D. Maclaren, T. Reilly and A. Lees), E & FN Spon, London, pp. 195-99.

6. Heck, H., Mader, A., Hess, G., Mucke, S., Muller, R. and Hollman, W. (1985) Justification of the 4-mmol/l lactate threshold. *Int. J. Sports Med.*, Vol. 6, pp. 117-30.

7. Scheen, A., Juchmes, J. and Cession-Fossion, A. (1981) Critical analysis of the "Anaerobic Threshold" during exercise at constant workloads. *Eur. J. Appl. Physiol.*, Vol. 46, pp. 367-77.

8. Tanaka, K. and Matsuura, Y. (1984) Marathon performance, anaerobic threshold, and onset of blood lactate accumulation. *J. Appl. Physiol.*, Vol. 57, pp. 640-43.

9. Craig, A.B., Skehan, P.L., Pawelczyk J.A. and Boomer, W.L. (1985) Velocity, stroke rate, and distance per stroke during elite swimming competition. *Med. Sci. Sports Exerc.*, Vol. 17, pp. 625-34.

10. Wakayoshi, K., Yoshida, T., Ikuta, Y., Mutoh, Y. and Miyashita, M. (1993) Adaptations to six months of aerobic swim training: Changes in velocity, stroke rate, stroke length and blood lactate. Int. J. Sports Med., Vol. 14, pp. 368-372.

ENERGETICS

23 COMPARISON OF PROPULSIVE FORCE IN FRONT CRAWL SWIMMING OBTAINED WITH TWO DIFFERENT METHODS

M.A.M. BERGER, A.P. HOLLANDER and
G. DE GROOT
Faculty of Human Movement Sciences, Vrije Universiteit,
Amsterdam, The Netherlands

Abstract
Propulsive forces during front crawl swimming using arms only were calculated on two different ways: based upon a kinematic analysis using 3D video analysis (Fp-3D) and based upon measurements of propulsive force on the MAD system (Fp-MAD). The two methods produced comparable values of propulsive force, although the values for Fp-MAD were lower in almost all cases. The mean difference between Fp-MAD and Fp-3D is 8 N, which is approximately 15%.
Keywords: front crawl swimming, propulsive force, 3D video analysis

1 Introduction

Direct measurement of propulsive forces during swimming is difficult due to the aquatic environment. To measure the propulsive forces a three dimensional kinematic analysis combined with data of drag and lift coefficients (Cd and Cl) derived from measurements in fluid laboratories was established by Schleihauf [1]. From video analysis an estimation of hand and forearm propulsive forces can be made, but validation of the calculated forces has only been done once: Hollander et al [2] compared the propulsive forces measured in two different ways: 1) hydrodynamic analysis based on underwater video registration of hand movements using Schleihauf's method, and 2) direct measurement of push-off forces using the MAD system (system for measuring active drag). Comparable values were found, although the MAD data was 10% higher. This discrepancy might be influenced by inaccuracies of Schleihauf's method: e.g., independent Cd and Cl values for hand and forearm, neglecting interaction effects between these two segments and a limited resolution. In the present study an increased resolution of the video system combined with the DLT-method was used for a more accurate determination of the orientation of hand and forearm. Further, Cd and Cl values determined for the combination of hand and forearm [3] were used. The resulting propulsive forces obtained by this improved 3D video analysis were compared with the forces from direct measurements by means of the MAD-system.

2 Methods

Three subjects, two male and one female swimmer of international level participated in a kinematic analysis and a MAD analysis. In both experiments the swimmers swam front crawl strokes in a 25 m pool using their arms only, their legs were supported and fixed together by a small buoy.

2.1 Kinematic analysis
Three-dimensional (3D) underwater videography was used to record the position of the hand and arm during a full stroke of one arm. The underwater pulling patterns of the right arm were filmed from the front, the right (2x) [4] and the bottom side using four gen-locked Panasonic video cameras operating at a speed of 50 frames per second. Two periscope systems [5] and an underwater housing were positioned to collect these three views of the arm strokes. Calibration took place with a reference frame of 1.0 x 1.0 x 2.0 meter. An overview of the set-up is given in figure 1.

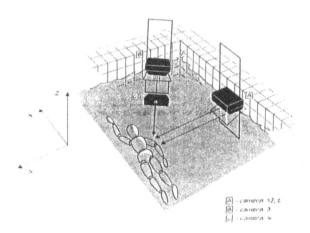

Fig. 1. Schematic overview of the experimental set-up

Motions and orientation of the hand were analyzed with help of black markers drawn on anatomical landmarks on hand and forearm, The landmarks were placed on the top of the third finger, the second and fifth metacarpophalangeal joint, the ulnar and radial side of the radiocarpal joint, the olecranon and on epicondylus radialis. Image co-ordinates were obtained manually at a sampling frequency of 50 Hz, and transformed to three-dimensional co-ordinates using the direct linear transformation (DLT) method.

Generated drag and lift forces by the hand and forearm were calculated according to the following equations:

$$Fd = 0.5r \ vhand2 \ AwCd \tag{1}$$
$$Fl = 0.5r \ vhand2 \ AwCl \tag{2}$$

where Fd = drag force (N), Fl = lift force (N), r = density of water, vhand = velocity of the hand (m*s-1), Aw = wet surface area (m2), Cd = coefficient of drag and Cl coefficient of lift. Cd and Cl were obtained in a previous study [3].

The velocity vhand was calculated from the marker on the fifth metacarpophalangeal joint (MCP5). The wet surface area Aw was estimated by taking the circumference of the arm every 2 cm along its length.

Cd and Cl are dependent on the orientation of the hand with respect to the direction of movement. According to Schleihauf [1], this direction is expressed by the angle of pitch (AP) and the sweep-back angle (SB). AP is the angle between the hand plane and the flow vector and SB is the orientation of the flow vector when projected on the hand plane. For a more detailed description the reader is referred to Berger et al. [3].

After calculating AP and SB it was possible to obtain the values of Cd and Cl and to calculate Fd and Fl. The propulsive force (Fp-3D) was calculated at each video frame according to:

$$Fp\text{-}3D = Fdx + Flx \tag{3}$$

where Fdx and Flx are respectively the drag and lift force in forward (x) direction. The mean propulsive force was calculated from the positive values of Fp-3D.

In order to calculate the mean swimming velocity during the stroke a marker was placed on the hip, and digitized when the left arm entered the water and half a stroke later, when the right arm entered the water. The displacement of the hip divided by the elapsed time resulted in an estimation of the velocity (vhip) during the stroke.

2.2 MAD system
The propulsive force delivered by the arms of the swimmers was also measured on the MAD-system (system to measure active drag) [6]. The MAD-system allowed the swimmer to push off from fixed pads at each stroke. These push-off pads were mounted 1.35 m apart on a 23 meter horizontal rod which was mounted at approximately 0.8 meter below the water surface in a swimming pool. At one end of the swimming pool the rod was connected to a force transducer. The push-off forces were processed and stored on disk using a microcomputer. To measure propulsive force and to establish the relation between propulsive force and swimming velocity, subjects were asked to swim 10 lanes

at 10 different velocities. For each lane the mean propulsive force and mean swimming velocity was calculated. These ten velocity-propulsive force data were least square fitted to the function:

$$Fp\text{-}MAD = Av^n \qquad (4)$$

where Fp-MAD represents propulsive force for swimming on the MAD-system, v swimming velocity and A a constant of proportionality.

To achieve the propulsive force at the swimming velocity performed during the kinematic measurements, vhip was put into equation 4. This results in a value for Fp-MAD which can be compared with the propulsive forces calculated from the kinematic analysis (Fp-3D).

3 Results

Figure 2 shows the propulsive force (Fp-3D) at each video frame for one subject during one stroke calculated from the kinematic analysis. This figure demonstrates that in the beginning of the stroke the propulsive force is negative, but a pull is delivered on the last 28 frames resulting in a mean Fp-3D of 21.97 N for this stroke.

In figure 3 the mean propulsive forces calculated from the kinematic analysis (Fp-3D) are plotted versus the propulsive forces derived from the MAD experiments (Fp-MAD). It can be seen that Fp-MAD is somewhat lower than Fp-3D, for almost all strokes. The mean difference between Fp-MAD and Fp-3D is 8 N, which is approximately 15%.

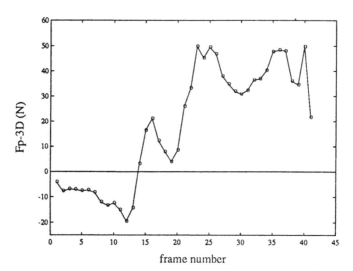

Fig. 2. Propulsive force (Fp-3D) for subject F1 during one stroke, at a velocity of 1.15 m.s-1.

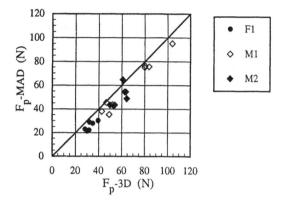

Fig. 3. Propulsive force calculated from the 3D experiments versus propulsive force as measured on the MAD-system (F1 = subject 1, M1 = subject 2, M2 = subject 3)

4 Discussion

In this study propulsive forces obtained from a 3D kinematic analysis were compared with direct measurements of the forces on the MAD-system. The MAD system enables the quantification of the propulsive force during front crawl swimming in a direct way. By comparing the propulsive force measured on the MAD-system with the propulsive forces calculated from a 3D video analysis the accuracy of this analysis can be established.

Figure 3 demonstrates that the two methods produce comparable values for the mean propulsive force, although for almost all strokes Fp-MAD is lower than Fp-3D. A possible explanation for this difference is that the velocity of MCP5 was put into equation 1 and 2. This velocity is higher than the velocity of the forearm, and will therefore result in an overestimation of the propulsive force from the kinematic analysis. In order to make the kinematic calculations more accurate, the velocity of hand and the velocity of the forearm had to be included in further calculations.

Differences between Fp-MAD and Fp-3D might also be due to difficulties in estimating the mean swimming velocity during the stroke from the video. The estimation of the mean swimming velocity was done by calculating vhip. It was difficult to measure vhip accurate, for two reasons. Firstly, the position of the hip could not be determined for the whole stroke, therefore only the position of the hip at left and right hand entry were analyzed. This resulted in a displacement in x position of the hip only based on two video frames, with a limited resolution. Secondly, the displacement in x position of the hip was divided by the number of frames from left hand entry to half a stroke later, right hand entry. The effect of differences in vhip are magnified in the calculation of Fp-3D by the exponent n (approx. 2) in equation 4. As a consequence, a deviation in vhip can lead to a large deviation in Fp-3D.

Despite the problems mentioned it can be concluded that the calculation of propulsive forces from 3D kinematic analysis results in a good estimation of propulsive forces used during swimming. In future experiments the results can be improved by a more accurate estimation of the combined hand and forearm velocity as well as the fluctuation in velocity of the body during actual swimming.

5 References

1. Schleihauf, R.E. (1979) A hydrodynamic analysis of swimming propulsion. *In: Swimming III*, (eds. J. Terauds and E.W. Bedingfield), University Park Press, Baltimore, pp. 70-109.
2. Hollander, A.P., Troup, J.P., Schleihauf, R.E.and Toussaint, H.M., (*submitted to J. of Biomechanics*). The determination of drag in front crawl swimming.
3. Berger, M.A.M, Groot, de G., and Hollander, A.P., (*in press, J. of Biomechanics*) Hydrodynamic lift and drag forces on human hand/arm models.
4. Payton, C.J., & Bartlett, R.M., (1993) A kinematic analysis of the breaststroke pulling patterns of national and international level swimmers. *Proc. of the XIVth ISB-congress*, Paris, 1012-1013.
5. Hay, J.G. and Gerot, J.T. (1991) Periscope systems for recording the underwater motions of a swimmer. *International Journal of Sports Biomechanics*, 7, 392-399.
6. Hollander, A.P., de Groot, G., van Ingen Schenau, G.J., Toussaint, H.M., de Best, H., Peeters, W., Meulemans, A., and Schreurs, A.W. (1986), Measurement of active drag during crawl arm stroke swimming. *Journal of Sport Sciences*, 4, 21-30.

Acknowledgment. We wish to thank Henk de Best and Rob van Lieshout for their technical support, and our students Johan Schalkwijk, Kirsten Bijker en Tanja Hogenhout for their cooperation in the process of data collection.

24 SPEED FLUCTUATIONS AND ENERGY COST OF DIFFERENT BREASTSTROKE TECHNIQUES

J.P. VILAS-BOAS
Porto University, Faculty of Sport Sciences, Porto, Portugal

Abstract
The purposes of this study were to: (i) compare hip speed fluctuations and swimming economy among three different breaststroke techniques: the flat style (FB), the undulated style (UB), and the new undulated style with overwater recovery of the arms (UOB); and (ii) study the relationships between these parameters. Subjects were 13 national top level swimmers, but for swimming economy tests, only 9 swimmers were studied. Swimming economy profiles for each of the three breaststroke techniques were assessed using net total oxygen consumption (VO_2) values and maximal net blood lactate concentrations after exertion. Speed fluctuation profiles were assessed through the photographic light trace of a pulse light device attached to the swimmer. After digitizing, pairs of values for time and speed were modelled using constrained polynomial regression procedures. Using the model, a transformed Strukhal number was calculated as an index of overall speed fluctuations. Results showed that for the speeds studied: (i) UOB was the least economical of the three breaststroke techniques studied; (ii) UOB implies higher speed fluctuations within a stroke cycle than FB and UB; and (iii) speed fluctuations and energy expenditure are correlated variables when intraindividual results are considered.
Keywords: Swimming, breaststroke, economy, energy cost, speed fluctuations

1 Introduction

Differences in average competition speed between breaststroke and more continuous techniques, such as front crawl, may be partially attributed to the less constant speed imposed by the technical characteristics of breaststroke swimming [1]. When swimming speed is not constant, the swimmer must deliver an extra power to overcome inertial forces, which should be reflected in the total energy output, and in the individual swimming performance potential. The theoretical relevance of swimming speed fluctuations within a stroke cycle, is very well documented in literature on swimming biomechanics, specially when breaststroke swimming is considered [1]. Nevertheless, to our knowledge, the relationship between swimming speed fluctuations and energy expenditure in swimming was not yet studied.

The purposes of this study were to: (i) compare hip speed fluctuations and swimming economy among three different breaststroke techniques: the flat style (FB), the undulated style (UB), and the new undulated style with overwater recovery of the arms (UOB); and (ii) study the relationships between these parameters.

2 Methods

Subjects were 13 well-trained national top level breaststroke swimmers. All of them participated in the speed fluctuations study, but the economy profiles and the relationship between parameters were studied only on 9 swimmers. Mean age was 15.8 (± 2.17) years, mean weight was 59.2 (± 9.37) kg, and mean height was 167.7 (± 7.64) cm. All swimmers were evaluated in the three breaststroke forms, and were previously trained to perform their non characteristic techniques.

The methodology for swimming economy assessment is described elsewhere [2]. Subjects performed a 3 x 200 m triangular protocol in each breaststroke technique, with a 30 min rest period between stages. Two stages were performed at submaximal speeds and the third stage of each testing session was a maximal effort. Total oxygen consumption (VO_2) at rest and per stage was directly measured using a *Sensormedics 2900* oxymeter, moved on a special chariot along the pool, and connected to the swimmer by a Toussaint's valve [3]. Ear-lob capillary blood samples were collected at rest and at 1, 3, 5, 7 and 10 min of recovery, and analysed for maximal blood [LA-] using an enzymatic photometric method (*Boehringer Mannheim*). Mean swimming speed per stage was determined through the mean time needed to cover the 10 central meters of the 25 m indoor swimming-pool. Net values of energy expenditure were obtained through the addition, divided by the exertion time, of the net total VO_2 values and maximal net blood [LA-] after exertion, transformed into VO_2 equivalents using a 2.7 $mlO_2 . kg^{-1} . mM^{-1}$ constant [4]. Individual and sample energy expenditure vs. swimming speed regressions for each of the three breaststroke techniques were determined. Differences between regression lines were tested using stepwise procedures with dummy variables.

Speed fluctuation profiles were assessed through a photo-optical method [5], using a extended exposure photographic light trace (*Canon* T70, 1000 ASA film) of a pulse light device placed in the waist of the swimmer, at a middle distance between the two hip joints. Swimmers performed 3 x 20 m in each one of the three breaststroke techniques, at a mean speed paced to be constant and close to the speed of each maximum 200 m trial of the economy tests.

After digitizing the photographic trace (*CalComp* table and *Sigma Scan* software), pairs of values for time (t) and speed (V) were modelled using 8 th degree polynomial regression procedures with two constraints: same first ($V_{t=0}$) and last ($V_{t=T}$) speed values of the stroke cycle and same first derivative values of speed in order of time in the same moments [6]. The model was obtained after translation of three consecutive cycles over the central one, allowing the determination of the best T value trough the best fit curve (higher r^2 value). The mean speed value for the stroke cycle was obtained through integration of the model for the cycle duration T. Using the model, $t_{(t1....,t4)}$ values for maximum (legs - V_2 - and arms - V_4 - actions) and minimum (legs recovery - V_1 - and transition between legs and arms actions - V_3) speed values during the stroke cycle were determined trough derivation. Integration and derivation of mathematical functions were performed through *PC-Matlab*, 3.13 software. A Strukhal (Sh) number [7], transformed for bimodal intracyclic speed fluctuations, was computed as a index of overall speed fluctuations within a stroke cycle:

$$Sh = \frac{\overline{V}_{(t=0,\ t=T)}}{(V_2 - V_1) + (V_4 - V_3)} \tag{1}$$

Individual Sh values of the 9 subjects sample were correlated with energy cost values ($mlO_2 . kg^{-1} . m^{-1}$) calculated for the same subjects, swimming at the same mean speed, using individual energy expenditure vs. swimming speed regression equations. Statistical procedures also included the computation of means and standard deviations and one-way ANOVA for repeated measures (Fisher PLSD).

3 Results

The economy profiles of the three breaststroke techniques presented in Fig. 1 point out that UOB was the least economic of the studied techniques. No significant difference was found between UB and FB. This tendency persisted when the 9 subjects sample was studied for the energy cost of locomotion (E). However, in this case the difference among undulated techniques was significant only for a 90% confidence interval.

As well as observed for the economy profiles, UOB was also the breaststroke technique that, for the mean swimming speeds studied, imposed the lowest Sh values (Fig. 1). This shows that this breaststroke technique was the one that imposed highest intracyclic speed fluctuations with respect to the mean swimming speed.

Overall correlation coefficient (r) between E and Sh was $r = - 0.168$. Individual correlation and determination (r^2) coefficients obtained between the two variables are presented in table 1. The mean value of the associated variance of both variables was 84.3%.

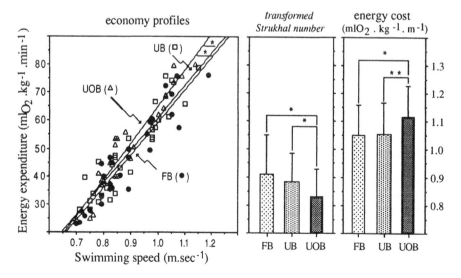

Fig. 1. Economy profiles, and mean and standard deviation values for transformed *Strukhal* number and for energy cost of each breaststroke technique: flat (FB), undulated (UB), and undulated style with overwater recovery of the arms (UOB). * ($p < 0.05$); ** ($p < 0.1$).($1\ lO_2 = 4.9$ kcal).

Table 1. Correlation (r) and determination (r^2) coefficients computed between Sh and E for each swimmer (A, ..., I).

	A	B	C	D	E	F	G	H	I
r	- 0.989	- 0.940	- 0.988	- 0.659	- 1	- 1	- 0.567	- 0.999	- 0.999
r^2	0.979	0.884	0.976	0.434	1	1	0.322	0.998	0.998

The mean values of the swimming speeds used to study Sh and E of the three breaststroke techniques were not significantly different ($p<0.05$): 1.06 (± 0.102) m . sec^{-1} for FB; 1.04 (± 0.120) m . sec^{-1} for UB; and 1.05 (± 0.100) m . sec^{-1} for UOB.

4 Discussion

The highest intra-cyclic speed fluctuations observed in the UOB when compared with FB, might seem to be a controversial result. In fact, previous results pointed out lowest speed fluctuations within a stroke cycle for undulated breaststroke techniques, when compared with the flat style [8]. Nevertheless, our results support Tourny's [9] idea that flat styles impose less intracyclic speed fluctuations than undulated ones.

The high mean swimming speed of the study of Colman & Persyn [8], and the relative slow-pace studied in this work (speeds lower than 200 m race pace), might contribute to explain the different findings. It is a well known characteristic of breaststroke, that increased speed changes technique synchronization, namely the time gap between the occurrence of maximum speeds associated to the leg kick and arm stroke [10]. This effect is produced by a increased superposition of the successive legs and arms actions, reducing a transition or a hypothetical gliding phase, and resulting in a less pronounced deceleration after V_2 and in higher V_3 values [11]. At submaximal speeds, identical to those we studied, it can be hypothesized that the swimmer performing the UOB can't reduce the power of the armstroke due to the need of the emersion of the upper limbs; to emerge the arms it is specially important to accelerate them during the insweep, which seem to be the most propulsive phase of the breaststroke arm action [8]. Doing so, the swimmer should increase the gliding phase, and increase speed fluctuations, in order to keep the pace with a submaximal speed.

High variations in swimming speed within a stroke cycle should impose an also high energy cost, since energy should be delivered to overcame inertial forces. This theoretically derived statement seems to be in accordance with a quick overview of Fig.1 results: the highest the energy cost, the highest the speed fluctuations, as shown by a lower Sh value. Nevertheless, the correlation found between both variables ($r = -0.168$) seems to be completely out of match with the previous arguments. On the other hand, individual r values (table 1) were amazingly high, revealing a mean value of 84.3% for the associated variance of both parameters.

The apparent discrepancy of sample and individual r values can be easily understood with a deep analysis on swimming bioenergetics. The work done while swimming is dependent on the mean swimming speed, the intracyclic speed fluctuations and the drag force [1]. Holmér [12] rose to evidence the relationship between the energy cost and the drag force. Meanwhile, the drag force that a swimmer should overcome at a given mean speed is widely variable and dependent on individual morphology and technique [13]. In accordance to the previous arguments, it must be expected that the energetic implications of a given velocity change should be strongly influenced by individual characteristics related with drag and with the efficiency of the different steps of chemical energy transformation [14].

5 Conclusions

Summarizing, the results of this study showed that, for the swimming speeds tested: (i) UOB was the least economic of the three breaststroke techniques studied; (ii) UOB implied higher speed fluctuations within a stroke cycle than FB and UB; and (iii) speed fluctuations and energy expenditure are correlated variables when intraindividual results are considered.

6 References

1. Nigg, B.M. (1983) Selected methodology in biomechanics with respect to swimming, in *Biomechanics and Medicine in Swimming*, (ed. A.P. Hollander, P.A. Huijing and G. de Groot), Human Kinetics Publishers, Champaign, Illinois, pp. 72-80.
2. Vilas-Boas, J.P. and Santos, P. (in press) Comparison of swimming economy in three breaststroke techniques, in *Medicine and Science in Aquatic Sports, Medicine and Sport Science*, Vol. 39, Karger, Basel.
3. Toussaint, H.M., Meulemans A., de Groot, G, Hollander, A.P., Schreurs, A.W. and Vervoorn, K (1987) Respiratory valve for oxygen uptake measurements during swimming. *Eur. J. Appl. Physiol.* , No. 56. pp. 363-366.
4. Di Prampero, P.E., Pendergast, D.R., Wilson, D.W., Rennie, D.W. (1978) Blood lactate acid concentrations in high velocity swimming, in *Swimming Medicine IV*, (eds. B. Eriksson and B. Furberg), University Park Press, Baltimore, pp. 249-261.
5. Vilas-Boas, J.P. (1992) A photo-optical method for the acquisition of biomechanical data in swimmers, in *ISBS'92 Proceedings*, (eds. R. Rodano, G. Ferrigno and G.C. Santambrogio), Edi.Ermes, Milano, pp. 142-145.
6. Vilas-Boas, J.P. (in press). A modelling method for discrete low sampling frequency temporal series on the evaluation of intracyclic swimming speed fluctuation. *ISBS'94 Proceedings*.
7. Kolmogorov, S.V. and Duplishcheva, O.A. (1992) Active drag, useful mechanical output and hydrodynamique force coefficient in different swimming strokes at maximal velocity. *J. Biomechanics*, Vol. 25, No. 3. pp. 311-318.
8. Colman, V., Persyn, U. (1991) *Diagnosis of the movement and physical characteristics leading to advice in breaststroke*. Continental Corse in Swimming for Coaches. FINA-COI-DSV, Gelsenkirshen.
9. Tourny, C. (1992) *Analyse des parametres biomechaniques du nageur de brasse de haut niveau*. Ph.D. Thesis, University of Montpellier, Montpellier.
10. Bober, T. and Czabanski, B. (1975) Changes in breaststroke techniques under different speed conditions, in *Swimming II*, (eds. J. P. Clarys and L. Lewillie), University Park Press, Baltimore, pp. 188-193.
11. Costill, D.L., Lee, G. and D'Acquisto, R.J. (1987) Video-computer assisted analysis of swimming technique. *J. Swim. Research*, Vol. 3, No. 2. pp. 5-9.
12. Holmér, I. (1974) Energy cost of arm stroke, leg kick and the whole stroke in competitive swimmers. *Eur. J. Appl. Physiol.*, No. 33. pp. 105-118.
13. Clarys, J.P. (1979) Human morphology and hydrodynamics, in *Swimming III*, (eds. J. Terauds and E. W. Bedingfield), University Park Press, Baltimore, pp. 3-41.
14. Troup, J.P. and Daniels, J.T. (1986) Swimming economy: an intruductory review. *J. Swim Research*, No. 2. pp. 5-9.

25 ENERGETIC EFFECTS OF VELOCITY AND STROKE RATE CONTROL IN NON-EXPERT SWIMMERS

D. CHOLLET
Centre d'Optimisation de la Performance Motrice, UFR-STAPS Montpellier, France

P. MORETTO, P. PELAYO and M. SIDNEY
Laboratoire d'Etude de la Motricite Humaine, Faculte des Sports, Lille, France

Abstract

The improving swimmer's skill characteristics pass from voluntary motor control (where conscious attention is required) to automatic control (where attention is not required but may be called on, leaving conscious mechanisms available for strategic purposes). What happens in the case of the moderately-skilled swimmer, particularly one who is working toward a peak skill level? From an energetic point of view, is swim performance under voluntary control more costly than that under automatic control?

Nine moderately-skilled adult swimmers (3 females, 6 males) whose performance time in the 400-m front crawl was 5 min 35 $\pm$ 8.5 s participated in 3 test sessions: 1) swim velocity (V) and stroke rate (SR) were self-selected by the subjects; 2) V was imposed; and 3) V and SR were imposed. In each session, heart rate (HR) was recorded and blood lactate concentration ([L]) was determined.

The principal finding was that although an increased energy cost was expected for the imposed V and SR trials, the two relevant parameters (HR and [L]) showed no increases, and indeed, some significant reductions.

Key words: energy cost, motor control, non-expert swimmers.

1 Introduction

The expert swimmer is characterized by a high level of performance with great stability in the management of racing parameters (a good distribution of velocity in the trials of a competitive meet, constancy of stroke rate and stroke length), indicating an excellent adaptation of technique and optimal energetic efficiency.

It appears that the notion of optimization is key to maximal efficiency. Indeed, there is an optimal relation between velocity and energy cost and also between stroke rate and stroke length. In order to achieve optimal ratios, adequate practice and highly complex motor control are necessary [1]. The acquisition of such highly-developed coordination by the expert is accomplished in two phases. The first phase requires the programming of a new structure of the elementary motor components of the system and the second requires the acquisition of automatic control of motor function necessary to reduce the energy cost; in this phase all superfluous movements are eliminated. The achievement of automatic control is characterized by the fluidity of the performance and the lowest possible cost to conscious attention (i.e., the capacity to do something else at the same time). The study of the characteristics of experts in tennis, swimming, and even piano show that this expertise is always linked to the achievement of automatic motor control. Logan's theory of automatic control [2] proposed that rapidity, lack of effort, autonomy, the lack of need for conscious thought, and direct access to memory are the characteristics of this mode of control. Indeed, beginners at a given task who are unable to rely on specific memory cannot control their actions in an automatic manner. They are constantly in a state of attentiveness, and thus of increased energy cost.

The aim of this study was to investigate the relation between energy expenditure and mode of control in terms of the relations that exist between velocity, stroke rate, and stroke length in non-expert swimmers who are in the process of developing automatic motor control.

2 Materials and Method

2.1 Subjects
Nine subjects (3 females and 6 males), students at the School of Physical Education in Lille, participated in this study. Mean age was 21.4 ± 5.25 years; mean height 174 ± 7 cm; mean weight 69.6 ± 9.38 kg and mean arm span 179 ± 8 cm. Their mean time for the 400-m freestyle was 5 min 35 ± 8.5 s.

2.2 Procedure
The three sessions were each composed of three trials: the 150-m crawl at slow, moderate and fast pace. A 4-min recovery period always separated each of the trials. An interval of 3-4 days separated the sessions, which were very specific:
- In the first session (S1), for each trial the velocity (V) and stroke rate (SR) were selected by the subject and the performance was recorded.
- In the second session (S2) for each trial, although SR remained self-selected, V was imposed. In order to do this, the swimmer was equipped with a luminous device connected to a velocity programmer. The V to be reproduced every 25 meters was in fact exactly the same as that selected by each swimmer in S1 (without the subjects being informed of this).
- In the third session (S3) and for each trial, in addition to the imposed V with the above-described procedure, SR was also imposed. This was done by means of an auditive device marking underwater the tempo corresponding to the imposed SR over the entire trial. The SR to be reproduced every 25 meters was exactly the same as that chosen by each swimmer in S1 (again without the subject being informed).

Data were recorded on video tapes.

During each session, heart rate (HR) was continuously recorded by a cardiofrequency meter and blood lactate concentration ([L]) was determined during the recovery period 3 min after every 150-m trial and 12 minutes following the last trial.

2.3 Data analysis
The data recorded over the course of the experiment were as follows:
- the 3 mean Vs ($m.s^{-1}$) (slow, moderate, fast) of each subject in each of the three sessions for a total of 9 values per subject,
- the three corresponding mean SRs ($cycles.min^{-1}$).

The physiological parameters which indicated the time course of energy cost were as follows:
- HR ($beats.min^{-1}$) was continuously recorded over the course of the experiment, allowing us to determine for each subject the mean HR of each trial, i.e., 9 values per subject, to which were associated 9 values of maximal HR and 9 values of minimal HR.
- [L] ($mmol.l^{-1}$) was measured at rest before each session, after each of the 3 trials, and at the end of each session, allowed us to study 15 values per subject.

Statistical analysis was conducted with the Wilcoxon non-parametric test for paired groups. Significance was fixed at $p < 0.05$ (*) and $p < 0.01$ (**).

3 Results

3.1 Stroke rate

The SRs of S1 and S2 were compared to determine the differences under the conditions of self-selected V and imposed V (Fig.1). Only one significant difference was noted ($p < 0.01$): for the fast pace, the self-selected SR in S1 (35.52 ± 3.21 cycles.min^{-1}) was higher than in S2 (34.07 ± 2.51). This corresponds to an increase in the stroke length (SL) from 2.07 ± 0.1 to 2.16 ± 0.09 m.cycle^{-1}.

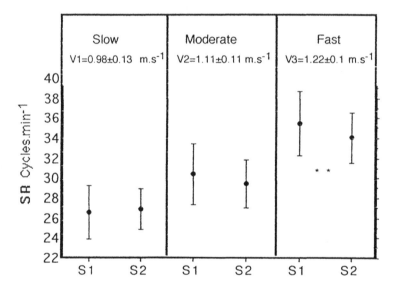

Fig. 1. Comparison of stroke rate (SR) between session 1 (S1), (self-selected velocity (V) and SR), and session 2 (S2), (imposed V and self-selected SR), for each of the 3 paces (slow, moderate, fast).

3.2 Physiological parameters

3.2.1 Heart rate

The mean HR values corresponding to 3x150-m (slow, moderate, and fast) were compared for each of the 3 sessions in order to identify the effects of control of V and of the associated control of V and SR (Fig.2).

No significant differences were found between mean HR whatever the swim pace. However, the maximal HR was significantly different ($p < 0.01$) with a maximal HR of 153.88 ± 14.82 beats.min1^{-}^{1} for the slow pace in S1 and 149.88 ± 13.98 beats.min^{-1} for the same pace in S3.

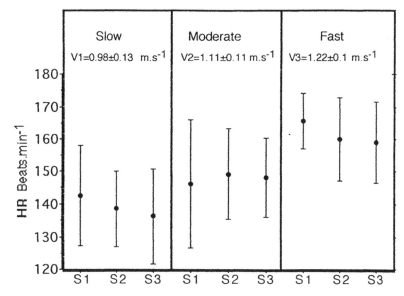

Fig. 2. Comparison of mean HR between session 1 (S1), with self-selected velocity (V) and stroke rate (SR); S2, with imposed V and self-selected SR; and S3, with both imposed V and SR. Comparisons were made at each pace (slow, moderate, fast).

3.2.2 Blood lactate concentration

The same comparisons as for HR were made for [L] with the addition of comparisons at rest and at the end of every session (Fig.3).

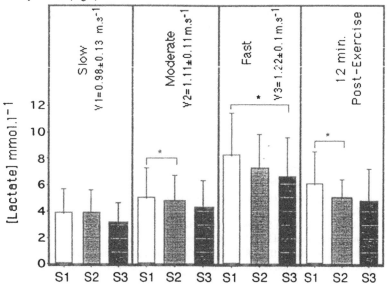

Fig. 3. Comparisons of blood lactate concentrations ([L]) between the three sessions (S1, S2, S3) during the three paces and at the end of each session.

No significant differences were calculated at rest or at the slow pace. Decreases ($p < 0.05$) were noted after the moderate pace between S1 (4.87 ± 2.14 mmol.l^{-1}) and S2 (4.37 ± 2.07 mmol.l^{-1}). Decreases ($p < 0.05$) were also noted after the fast pace between S1 (7.94 ± 3.25 mmol.l^{-1}) and S3 (6.64 ± 3.41 mmol.l^{-1}). During the final recovery period, this decrease was confirmed ($p < 0.05$) between S1 (5.91 ± 2.65 mmol.l^{-1}) and S2 (4.47 ± 1.66 mmol.l^{-1}).

4 Discussion and Conclusion

It is well known that energy cost increases with increases in velocity [3] and it has been shown that in swimming stroke length is also a factor which influences the energy cost [4;5].

Two modes of control of complex motor function, i.e., automatic and voluntary, have been distinguished [6]. Whereas the automatic mode is characterized by a non-required central capacity, high performance level, low conscious involvement (although conscious attention may be called upon) and low effort, the voluntary mode is the converse, characterized by a required central capacity, low performance level (except if the task is easy), high conscious involvement and enormous effort. In other words, one would expect to observe increased energy cost when the swimmer must control his velocity and stroke rate. On the contrary, however, our energetic parameters had a tendency to decrease. Although heart rate did not overall differ, lactate concentrations decreased.

During the control of performance, the information processed can be of two types: intrinsic (inherent to the task, e.g., tactile, proprioceptive) or extrinsic (that which is added, e.g., advice and instructions of the coach, chronometry, video, etc.). This information can be delivered during action (the notion of leaded performance) or after action (the notion of feedback). It seems for our non-expert but confirmed swimmers that the information on velocity or stroke rate, provided by external means, played more of a leading role instead of the constraining role that we expected. This hypothesis was supported by the decrease in stroke rate, and thus the corresponding increase in stroke length, leading one to assume a better adaptation of technique.

It is difficult to think that this study could invalidate the theories of motor control showing a higher energy cost for the mode of voluntary control. On the contrary, we show that an external control of velocity or stroke rate does not prevent the acquisition of an automatic mode of control. The effects of motor learning during the three sessions and the contribution of guiding information from the exterior explain for this population the decrease in energy cost during these trials.

5 References

1.   Schmidt, R.A. (1988) *Motor Control and Learning,* Human Kinetics Publishers, Champaign, Il.
2.   Logan G.D. (1985) Skill and automaticity: relation, implication and future directions. *Canadian Journal of Psychology.*, Vol. 39, pp. 367-386.
3.   Holmér, I. (1972) Oxygen uptake during swimming in man. *Journal of Applied Physiology,* Vol. 33, pp. 502-509.
4.   Costill, D.L., Maglischo, E.W. and Richardson, A.B. (1992) Physiological Evaluation, in *Handbook of Sports Medicine and Science Swimming.* Blackwell Scientific Publications, Oxford.
5.   Keskinen, K.L. (1993) *Stroking Characteristics of Front Crawl Swimming.* Studies in Sport, Physical Education and Health 31. University of Jyväskylä.
6.   Schneider, W. and Shiffrin, R.M. (1977) Controlled and automatic human information processing I. Detection search and attention. *Psychological Review*, Vol. 84, pp. 1-66.

26 ENERGY METABOLISM DURING SPRINT SWIMMING

S. RING*, A. MADER*, W. WIRTZ**, K. WILKE**
*Inst. for Cardiology and Sportsmedicine and **Inst. of Aquatic Sports, German Sports University, Cologne, Germany

Abstract

The present investigation is an attempt to give a view of the complexity of energy metabolism in sprint swimming with the help of a *differential equation simulation model*. From this computer simulation it becomes clear, that the glycolytic pathway play an important role early in 50 m sprint swimming. This depends on the quick PCr-depletion to continue the swim in maximal speed. The role of VO_2 for 50 m shall not be underestimated, too.

Keywords: energy metabolism, sprint swimming

Introduction

In 1988 at the Olympic Games in Seoul sprint swimming (50 m crawl) became part of the olympic programm. This discipline is characterized by a peak power output approximately between 9.0 - 11.6 W/kg body weight (BW) [13] and a high developed technical ability. Measuring of the energy metabolism during free sprint swimming was not often researched until yet, mainly because of methodical difficulties. In this study we tried to establish the contribution of the aerobic and anaerobic demand during free sprint swimming by determining post peak oxygen uptake (VO_2), maximal post blood lactic acid concentration (La) and swimming performance (velocity). The experimental data were put into the simulation model of Mader (1984) [8]. This model assumes, that the dynamic changes of the phosphorylation-state of the high energy phosphate system, as a result of contraction, the adjustment of the rate of glycolysis and oxidative

phosphorylation as well as lactic accumulation in muscle compartment and distribution from muscle to a passive compartment, could be calculated by a system of differential equations [8,9].
The purpose of this study is :

1)   to figure out an approach of the pattern of energy supply in free sprint swimming,
2)   to use experimental data for recalculating the dynamic of energy supply during sprint basded on the differential equation system.

2 Method

Twelve club swimmers in the age of 23.3 ±3.3 yr, 186.1 ±6.9 cm height and 80.9 ±8.9 kg body weight volunteered in the present investigation. They were fully informed about the experiment before written consent was obtained. To accentuate the differences in energy supply in sprint swimming between a sprinter and a long distance swimmer, data were estimated for them, too. The anthropometrical data of the sprinter were 30 yr, 193 cm, 93.6 kg and of the non-sprinter 25 yr, 178 cm and 69.5 kg.
   At first they completed 15, 25 and 50 m crawl in maximal speed starting from the competition postition. Between each sprint was a rest period of 15 - 30 min. Blood samples were taken after performance in the 1.,2.,3.,4.,5.,6.,7.,12.,15. and 20. min from the hyperhaemizised earlobe for determining maximal La. Data are shown in table 1. The 15 and 25 m were swum without any breath, whereas in the 50 m two breaths were permitted. Immediately after each distance the swimmer had to hold the breath until a three valve respiratory mask was connected to his face. Afterwards the swimmer was wrapped into cloth and gas exchange were measured with an open spirometric system during the whole rest period in the sitting position. After two days the two distance test (2x400m crawl) [10] was swum to ascertain the aerobic performance level, by measuring La in the same way as described before.

Table1.   Data of the field tests (mean and ± sd)

Average (n=12)	15m	25m	50m	400m
v (m/s)	2.4/(±0.1)	2.1 (±0.1)	1.9 (±0.1)	1.3 (±0.7)
t (s)	6.3 (±0.4)	11.9 (±0.7)	26.5 (±1.6)	308.6 (±16.7)
La (mmol/l)	3.1 (±0.9)	5.6 (±1.5)	9.1 (±2.7)	7.7 (±2.8)
VO_2(ml/kg*min) [1]	33.3 (±4.2)	42.7 (±5.2)	50.7 (±3.7)	[49.4] [2]
Nonsprinter				
v (m/s)	2.2	2	1.7	1.3
t (s)	6.9	12.8	29.5	315
La (mmol/l)	2.7	3.8	5.7	4.2
VO_2(ml/kg*min) [1]	33.2	35.1	46.6	[45.1] [2]
Sprinter				
v (m/s)	2.6	2.2	2	1.2
t (s)	5.8	11.2	24.7	341.9
La (mmol/l)	3.7	7.2	12.3	10.5
VO_2(ml/kg*min) [1]	29.5	34.4	44.5	[43.5] [2]

([1] *peak oxygen uptake,* [2] *result of the simulation*)

For the simulation, parameters of the total adenine and phosphate pool, of glycolysis and the oxidative phosphorylation were supposed (Tab.2), based on published muscle biopsies and ^{31}PNMR-method measured data [2,14,18]. All data were determined for muscle weight (MW), 33% active muscle space and 48% water space of body volume. The reconversion factor for body weight (BW) amounts 0.33 [8,9]. From this we got an approach of the percentage of VO_2max, of the power output (W/kg BW) and of the contribution of the three energy systems, which correspond with the measured VO_2 (ml/kg BW * min) and La (mmol/l).

Table 2.   Assumed simulation parameters

	Average	Nonsprinter	Sprinter
PCr (mmol/kg MW)	21	21	21
Cr (mmol/kg MW)	9	9	9
ATP (mmol/kg MW)	5.98	4.99	5.98
ADP (mmol/kg MW)	0.043	0.036	0.043
VLa (mmol/l*s MW)	0.75	1.0	1.0
VO_2 (ml/kg *s MW)	2.9	3.0	2.65
VO_2 max (l/min BW)	4.645	4.098	4.932

No difference was made between the assumed phosphocreatine concentration (PCr) of the average group, the sprinter and non-sprinter. To distinguish between short and long distance swimmers adenosinetriphosphate concentration (ATP), maximal lactic building rate (VLa) and maximal oxygen uptake (VO_2max) were modified.

3 Results

Table 3 represents the results of the simulation of the whole group, the non-sprinter and sprinter.

Table 3.   Results of the simulation

Average (n=12)	15m	25m	50m	400m
W/kg BW	21.5	17.3	12.4	5.8
%VO$_2$ max (%)	58	62	74	86
VO$_2$ (l/min BW)	2.69	2.88	3.44	3.90
Nonsprinter				
W/kg BW	18.2	12.4	8.3	4.0
%VO$_2$ max (%)	54	68	70	76
VO$_2$ (l/min BW)	2.21	2.79	2.87	3.12
Sprinter				
W/kg BW	21.5	20.6	20.0	4.0
%VO$_2$ max (%)	56	60	74	83
VO$_2$ (l/min BW)	2.76	2.96	4.91	4.09

The 400 m VO$_2$-values of the two distance test (Tab.1), which were determined from the simulation data, agree well with other published data [4,11]. All data were converted into body weight (BW). The energy contribution for the whole group for 50 m crawl amounted to 35.2% alactic, 43.0% lactic and 21.8% aerobic. For 400 m crawl a percental distribution of 5.4 alactic to 17.2 lactic to 77.4 aerobic was detected. The non-sprinter shows a larger aerobic part for 50 and 400 m (35.0 : 35.9 : 29.1 and 4.4 : 9.1 : 86.5) than the average and the sprinter (22.5 : 59.7 : 17.8 and 6.8 : 14.2 : 76.0). Figure 1 shows the diffferences in energy metabolism during 50 m between the long-distance swimmer (a) and the sprinter (b).

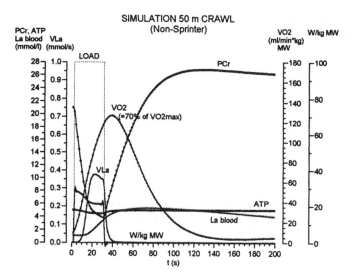

Fig. 1a.   Simulation of the non-sprinter

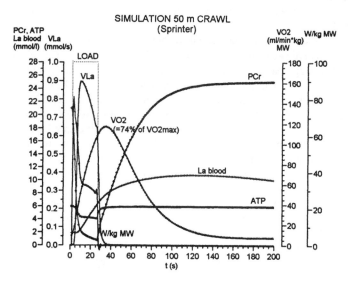

Fig. 1b. Simulation of the sprinter

Depending on the simulation set and swim time the simulation was performed by choosing a power output, which lead to the measured experimental La and VO_2, expressed in percent of VO_2 max (see table 1, 2 and figure 1).

4 Discussion

In reality the power output (W/kg BW) at 50 m of the sprinter, respectively 24.7 s, seems to be to high as compared with data of Olbrecht [13], who established a energy demand equation for constant velocity load. But the established output of this present study is an absolute one, therefore mean power output has to be determined, which amounts 13.5 W/kg BW for the sprinter and 7.8 W/kg BW for the non-sprinter. The data of the non-sprinter fit more to other published results of same exercise duration and maximal intensity, because a more slight decrease in power output (W/kg) was estimated as seen in figure 1a [5,17]. The difference between their power will be larger, if the training adaptions in the FTa-F for the sprinter were taken into account [1] and the VLa of the non-sprinter will be lowered.

The approximations of the whole group mean power output of 5.8 W/kg BW for 400 m as well as 3 l/min VO_2 at 4.0 mmol/l La and 1.3 m/s mean swimming velocity of the non-sprinter, representing 76 % VO_2max. This agrees also with published results [4,11,13]. The 400 m performance of the sprinter seems to be to small, but the real measured high La-level indicates a moderate developed aerobic capacity. So that a part of the oxidative metabolic capacity could only be used in case of a higher lactate production rate.

The simulation example (Fig. 1a and b) shows, that already after 5.8 - 6.3 s (first 15 m) a high glycolytic activation can be recognized, because of the relatively high La (≈ 3 mmol/l). This large participation of glycolysis, especially for the sprinter, expressed in 59.7 % of enery contribution, is necessary for rephosphorylating PCr, to keep ATP high, to continue work. These results agree well with other fingings [6,15]. Hirvonen et al. (1987) also pointed out, that after short supramaximal exercise (100 m sprint) a high lactic acid concentration and considerable decrease in running speed were noticed after 50 m run [3]. It seems possible to ascertain the PCr-content form the area of the post exercise oxygen uptake to resting level, by fitting the experimental curves with a varation of PCr of the muscle So that the VO_2 -curves in fiure 1 show a minimal difference to the experimental measured ones.

Another interesting finding of the presented data is, that the aerobic energy supply during 50 m sprint swimming shall not be underestimated. From the simulation we estimated 17.8 - 29.1 % aerobic contribution, whereas the aerobic part for 15 m was about 3 - 5 %. Because of reduced breathing the estimated aerobic contribution maybe was covered mainly by a decrease in oxygen-myoglobin depots [2,16].

In conclusion it has to be pointed out, that common views of energy supply for 50 m sprint swimming, 50% alactic : 48% lactic : 2% aerobic [12], underestimate the early activation of glycolysis and the aerobic contribution.

5 References

1. Costill, D.L. (1978) *Adaptations in Skeletal Muscle during Training for Sprint and Endurance Swimming.* In: B. Eriksson, B. Furberg: Swimming Medicine IV, Baltimore, pp. 233-248.
2. Hermansen, L. (1981) *Muscular Fatigue During Maximal Exercise of Short Duration.* In: P.E. DiPrampero, J. Porrtmans (eds.): Physiological chemistry of exercise, Medicine Sport, Vol. 13, 45-52.
3. Hirvonen, J., Rehunen, S., Rusko, H., Härkonen, M. (1987) *Breakdown of High-Energy Phosphate Compounds and Lactate Accumulation during Short Supramaximal Exercise.* Eur. J. Appl. Physiol., Vol. 56, pp. 253-259.
4. Holmer, I. (1974) *Physiology of Swimming Man.* Acta Physiol. Scand., Suppl. 407, pp. 1-53.
5. Jacobs, I., Tesch, P.A., Bar-Or, O., Karlsson, J., Dontan, R. (1983) *Lactate in Human Skeletal Muscle after 10 and 30 s of Supramaximal Exercise.* J. Appl. Physiol.: Respirat.Environ.Exercise Physiol. Vol. 55, No. 2, pp. 365-367.
6. Karlsson, J. (1971*) Muscle ATP, CP and Lactate in Submaximal and Maximal Exercise.* In: B. Pernow, B. Saltin: Muscle Metabolism During Exercise, New York, pp. 383-393.
8. Mader, A. (1984) *Eine Theorie zur Berechnung der Dynamik und des steady state von Phosphorylierungszustand und Stoffwechselaktivität der Muskelzelle als Folge des Energiebedarfs.* Habilitation, Köln.
9. Mader, A., Heck, H. (1986*) A Theory of the Metabolic Origin of „Anaerobic Threshold".* Int. J. Sports Med. Vol. 7, pp. 45-65.
10. Mader, A., Heck, H., Hollmann, W. (1976) *Evaluation of Lactic Acid Anaerobic Energy Contribution by Determination of Postexercise Lactic Acid Concentration of Ear Capillary Blood in Middle-distance Runners and Swimmers.* In: F. Landing., W. Orban (eds.): Exercise Physiology, Florida, pp. 187-199.
11. Madsen, O. (1982) *Untersuchungen über Einflußgrößen auf Parameter des Energiestoffwechsels beim freien Kraulschwimmen.* Dissertation, Köln.
12. Maglischo, E.W. (1993) *Swimming Even Faster.* Mountain View, California, p.21.
13. Olbrecht, J. (1989) *Metabolische Beanspruchung bei Wettkampfschwimmern unterschiedlicher Leistungsfähigkeit.* Dissertation, Brüssel.

14.   Sahlin, K., Harris, R.C., Hultman, E. (1975) *Creatine Kinase Equilibrium and Lactate Content Compared with Muscle pH in Tissue Samples Obtained after Isometric Exercise.* Biochem. J. Vol. 152, pp. 173-180.

15.   Sahlin, K., Edström, L., Sjöholm, H., Hultman, E. (1981) *Effects of Lactic acid accumulation and ATP decrease on muscle tension and relaxation.* Am. J. Physiol. Vol. 9, pp. C121-C126.

16.   Saltin, B., Essen, B. (1971) *Muscle Glycogen, Lactate, ATP and CP in Intermittent Exercise.* In: B. Pernow, B. Saltin: Muscle Metabolism During Exercise, New York, pp. 419-424.

17.   Seresse, O., Lortie, G., Bouchard, C., Boulay, M.R. (1988*) Estimation of the Contribution of the Various Energy Systems During Maximal Work of Short Duration.* Int. J. Sports Med. Vol. 9, pp. 456-460.

18.   Spriet, L.L. (1989) *ATP Utilization and Provision in Fast-Twich Skeletal Muscle during Tetanic Contractions.* Am. J. Physiol. Vol. 257, pp. E595-E605.

27 DETERMINANTS OF ENERGY COST OF FRONT CRAWL AND BACKSTROKE SWIMMING AND COMPETITIVE PERFORMANCE

F. ALVES, J. GOMES-PEREIRA and F. PEREIRA
Faculty of Human Movement, Lisbon, Portugal

Abstract
The purpose of this study was to investigate the relationships between swimming economy and selected body dimensions, stroking characteristics, intracycle body velocity variation and performance. Twelve well-trained male swimmers participated in this study. Every swimmer performed 3 x 250 m submaximal swims, progressive intensity, and a 400 m maximal swim. Oxygen uptake was measured from the expired air collected during the first 20 seconds of recovery, using the retroextrapolation method. A swimming economy profile was determined for each subject. Oxygen uptake measured after the maximal swim was considered to be the $\dot{V}O_2$ peak for each swimmer in that stroke. Swimmers were filmed underwater (sagital plane) during the 400 m swim to measure intracycle hip velocity variation. Every swimming effort was filmed for the assessment of stroke rate and effective velocity. Energy cost of backstroke showed a strong correlation with body dimensions, especially height and arm span. In both strokes, O_2 uptake at the velocity of 1.3 m.s^{-1} was inversely associated with best performance in the 200 and 400 m. No significant relationships were found between stroke cycle characteristics and energy cost at any velocity, but intracycle velocity variation amplitude of backstroke was positively correlated to energy cost at 1.1 and 1.2 m.s^{-1}.
Keywords: Backstroke, Body Size, Front Crawl, Oxygen Uptake, Performance, Stroke Cycle.

1 Introduction

Swimming economy is the energy cost associated with a given velocity of displacement. A lower energy cost for submaximal paces and a faster maximum swimming speed are advantages that result from a better swimming economy. The inter-individual variation of energy cost is usually large and is thought to depend mainly on technical ability [1]. Propelling efficiency, more than mechanical efficiency, seems to determine the slope of the economy line [2] and when propelling efficiency is high, the swimmers have large distances per stroke. This fact induced Costill et al. [3] to define a "stroke index", the product of swimming velocity and distance per stroke, to evaluate indirectly swimming economy. Other factors like body dimensions, body mass and buoyancy have also been shown to affect energy cost of swimming [3,4,5,6,7].

Few studies have focused on the energy cost of backstroke swimming [8, 9, 10]. Most of what has been investigated on this subject refers to front crawl and breaststroke. The purpose of the present study was to investigate the relationships between swimming economy in backstroke and front crawl swimming and selected body dimensions, stroking characteristics, intracycle velocity variation and performance.

2 Methods

Twelve well trained male swimmers participated in this study (age: 17.8 ± 1.8 years, height: 178.5 ± 6.1 cm, body mass: 67.6 ± 6.6 kg, and % adipose tissue: 7.6 ± 2.0). Testing protocol consisted of 3 submaximal 300 swims progressive intensity (65, 75 and 85 % of maximal velocity for that distance) and 1 x 400 maximal swim. Oxygen uptake was measured using the retroextrapolation method [11]. Every swimmer was told to hold his breath in the last arm stroke before touching the wall. As soon as he stopped swimming, a rubber mouthpiece and a nose clip were fitted to his face and he should begin to exhale in a normal way. The expired gas sample was collected during the first 20 seconds of recovery in a Douglas bag and then analysed for O_2 and CO_2 contents using a electronic gas analyser (Erich Jaeger, Germany), calibrated with gases of known concentrations. Volumes were measured with a mechanical gas meter (Wright, England) and values converted to STPD conditions. Correction of the recovery values was made following Costill et al.[3].Oxygen uptake measured after the maximal swim was considered to be the $\dot{V}O_2$ peak for each swimmer. Arterialised blood samples were collected after the last swimming bout, for the determination of blood lactate concentration. Swimmers were free of equipment and were instructed to keep a constant pace in each swim, following a light tracer. An exponential regression technique was used to describe the relation between swimming speed and rate of metabolism [12]. The $\dot{V}O_2$ / swimming speed relationship estimated for each subject was considered to be his swimming economy profile. The cost of transport, expressed in $J.m^{-1}$, [13] was calculated from each $\dot{V}O_2$ individual regression line at 1.1, 1.2, 1.3 and 1.4 $m.s^{-1}$ in front crawl and at 1.1, 1.2 and 1.3 m.s⁻¹ in backstroke. Cost per stroke was calculated for the same velocities dividing the oxygen demand by the stroke rate.

The swimmers were filmed underwater during the 400 swim with a video camera (30 Hz), fixed from the wall, 6 m from the swimmer, perpendicular to the direction of swimming and 20 cm underwater. The intracycle velocity curves in backstroke and front crawl were obtained by numerical treatment of data from the hip displacement in the last lap of 25 m and evaluated by a video analysing system. In spite of the known differences between intracycle velocity measured at the center of gravity or at the hip, Maglischo et al. [14] have proposed that the horizontal velocity of the hip can be used as a tool for technical evaluation because the velocities of the hip and center of gravity follow similar patterns in the four competitive strokes. Every swimming effort was filmed for the assessment of stroke rate and velocity. The effective velocity sustained at each stage was measured over 15 m within two points 5 m from each end of the pool, to eliminate the influence of the turn. Distance per stroke was then estimated by simple arithmetic calculations. Anthropometric measurements were made following standard procedures [15].

Best performances for the 100, 200, 400 and 1500 m swims were taken from official competitions that took place the month before or after the testing measurements.

All data are expressed as means ± S.D.. Student's t-test was performed to evaluate the difference in energy cost between front crawl and backstroke. Coefficients of variation (SD.mean⁻¹.100) were calculated for intracycle hip velocity. Correlations performed were Pearson Product Moment. Statistical significance was accepted at the level: $p < 0.05$.

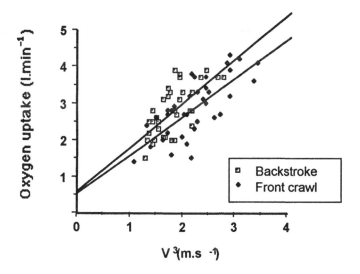

Figure 1. Energy cost and swimming velocity in front crawl and backstroke.

3 Results

$\dot{V}O_2$ (l.min⁻¹) increased linearly with the cubed value of swimming velocity following the equations $\dot{V}O_2 = 0.617+1.199V^3$ (r=0.68) for backstroke and $\dot{V}O_2 = 0.556+1.041V^3$ (r=0.74) for front-crawl swimming (Fig. 1). $\dot{V}O_2$ peak (l.min⁻¹) and lactate concentration (mmol.l⁻¹) were 4.13±0.44 and 11.94±1.51 in front-crawl and 3.91±0.39 and 9.68±2.23 in backstroke, respectively. $\dot{V}O_2$ peak was reached at a velocity of 1.4 m.s⁻¹ and 1.29 m.s⁻¹, in front crawl and backstroke, respectively. Intensity levels chosen for analysis of swimming economy corresponded to 79, 86, 93 and 100 % of critical velocity in front crawl and 85, 93 and 101 % in backstroke.

The cost of transport of both strokes increased as swimming velocity increased (Fig. 2), the difference between front crawl and backstroke becoming larger as velocity got higher.

Energy cost per stroke of backstroke showed a strong correlation with body dimensions, especially height and arm span (r = -.78 and r = -.70, respectively). In this stroke, $\dot{V}O_2$ peak was positively associated with weight and chest transverse area. In front crawl, the correlations between cost per stroke and body dimensions were weaker than in backstroke but showed the same tendency.

In both strokes, O_2 uptake at the velocity of 1.3 m.s⁻¹ was inversely associated with performance in the 400 m. In backstroke, the strongest correlations were found between the best time in the 200 m event and the cost per cycle at 1.3 m.s⁻¹. In front crawl cost per stroke at 1.3 m.s⁻¹ was also correlated to the 1500 m event. There were no significant relationships between performance and the $\dot{V}O_2$ peak in both strokes. No significant relationships were found between stroke characteristics and energy cost at any velocity, but intracycle velocity variation amplitude was positively correlated to energy cost at 1.1 and 1.2 m.s⁻¹ in backstroke.

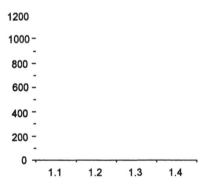

Figure 2. Cost of transport variation with velocity in front crawl and backstroke swimming.

4 Discussion

The early researchers who studied the energy cost of swimming at various velocities [16] indicated that these two variables were associated in an exponential manner. More recently, Lavoie and Montpetit [17] concluded that studies where a curvilinear association was observed suffered from several inaccuracies such as not having all the subjects swimming the entire range of velocities [5], calculation of energy expenditure additioning oxygen consumption during swimming to the oxygen debt actually measured or estimated from blood lactate concentrations. The linear regression technique has been used so far by several researchers. However, theoretically, power output increases with the cubed value of velocity, as can be deduced from the power equation of swimming, since it is assumed that drag has a quadratic relation with velocity. This was experimentally confirmed by Hollander et al. [12] in a swimming flume. In this study, the extrapolation of energy demand at higher velocities, as well as intercept values of the regression equations, were more realistic when exponential relation was used. The mean value of "r" was also higher, meaning that is the exponential extrapolation model that gives more accurate and reliable results.

The increase of cost of transport with velocity was predictable, since body drag, the main determinant factor on the energy cost of swimming, has a quadratic relationship with velocity. Moreover, propelling efficiency seems to decrease with velocity [18], what may explain further this occurrence. It has been reported that the specific energetic cost of backstroke swimming might be about 11 % greater than that of front crawl [10]. In our study the difference was more important, ranging from 16 % for a velocity of 1.1 m.s^{-1} to 32 % to a swimming velocity of 1.3 m.s^{-1}. The explanation for this discrepancy may rely in the fact that these group of swimmers were, in average, less proficient in backstroke than in front crawl, what could be easily confirmed by their race performance times.

Taller swimmers seemed to be more economical at submaximal velocities and arm span is one physical characteristic that may indicate what swimmers have a better improvement potential, probably because it propitiates a better propelling efficiency. These results are in agreement with what has been reported for backstroke swimming [9].

Contrarily to previous studies where the energy spent in accelerating the body in front and back crawl seemed to be negligible [8], we found a positive correlation between intracycle horizontal velocity fluctuation measured at the hip and energy cost at submaximal velocities. The higher energy cost for the same velocity range observed in backstroke was previously reported [8, 10] and is mainly due to less favourable mechanical conditions. This is confirmed by the higher intracycle velocity variation measured in backstroke than in front crawl, since every change in velocity results in an increase in the amount of work the swimmer must do. In backstroke also exists usually a stronger participation of the kick either for direct propulsive purposes or for balance of body position in the water to decrease drag, which results in a higher oxygen uptake because more muscle mass is put to work.

One of the main findings of our study is that we confirmed, after Smith et al. [9], that oxygen demand at maximal and submaximal velocities seems to be a good indicator of race performance in middle and long distance events and should be considered as an important tool for the evaluation and advise in training.

5 References

1.   Toussaint, H.M. (1992) Performance determining factors in front crawl swimming, in *Biomechanics and Medicine in Swimming - Swimming Science VI*, (eds. D. Maclaren, T. Reilly and A. Lees), E and FM Spon, London, pp. 13-32.

2.   Toussaint, H.M. (1990) Differences in propelling efficiency between competitive and triathlon swimmers. *Medicine and Science in Sports and Exercise*, Vol. 22 No.3, pp. 409-415.

3.   Costill D.L., Kovaleski, J., Porter, D., Kirwan, J., Fielding R. and King, D. (1985) Energy expenditure during front crawl swimming: predicting success in middle distance events. *International Journal of Sports Medicine*, Vol. 6, pp.266-270.

4.   Monpetit, R.R., Lavoie, J.-M. and Cazorla, G.A. (1983) Aerobic energy cost of swimming the front crawl at high velocity in international class and adolescent swimmers, in *International Series on Sports Sciences: Vol. 14: Biomechanics and Medicine in Swimming* , (eds. Hollander, P.; P. Huijing e G. deGroot), Human Kinetics, Champaign, pp. 228-234.

5.   Pendergast, D.A., diPrampero, P., Craig, A.B., Wilson, D.R. and Rennie, D.W. (1978) - Energetics of locomotion in man, in Exercise Physiology, (eds. F. Lery and W. A. R. Orban), Symposia Specialists Inc., Miami, pp. 61-70.

6.   Monpetit, R.R., Smith, H. and Boie, G. (1988) Topic report: swimming economy, how to standardize the data to compare swimming proficiency. *Journal of Swimming Research*, Vol. 4, No. 1, pp. 5-8.

7.   Chatard, J.C., Collomp, C., Maglischo, E. and Maglischo, C. (1990) Swimming skill and stroking characteristics of front crawl swimmers. *International Journal of Sports Medicine*, Vol. 11, No.2, pp.156-161.

8.   Holmér, I. (1974) Physiology of swimming man. *Acta Physiologica Scandinava*, Suppl. 407.

9.   Smith, H., Monpetit, R.R. and Perrault, H. (1988) The Aerobic demand of backstroke swimming and its relation to body size, stroke technique and performance. *European Journal of Applied Physiology*, Vol. 58, pp. 182-188.

10.   Klentrou, P.P. and Monpetit, R. R. (1992) Energetics of backstroke swimming in males and females. *Medicine and Science in Sports and Exercise*, Vol. 24, No. 3, pp. 371-375.
11.   Monpetit, R.R., Leger, L.A., Lavoie, J.M. and Cazorla, G.A. (1981) $\dot{V}O_2$ peak during free swimming using the backward extrapolation of the O_2 recovery curve. *European Journal of Applied Physiology*, Vol. 47, pp. 385-395.
12.   Hollander, A.P., Troup, J.P. and Toussaint, H.M. (1990) Linear vs. exponential extrapolation in swimming research (abs), in *Abstracts of the Sixth International Symposium on Biomechanics and Medicine in Swimming*, Liverpool Polytechnic. Liverpool.
13.   diPrampero, P.E. (1986) The Energy cost of human locomotion on land and in water. *International Journal of Sports Medicine*, Vol. 7, pp. 55-72.
14.   Maglischo, E.W.; Maglischo, C.M. and Santos, T.R. (1987) The relationship between the forward velocity of the center of gravity and the forward velocity of the hip in the four competitive strokes. *Journal of Swimming Research*, Vol.3, No.2, pp.11-17
15.   Lohman, T.G., Roche, A.F. and Martorell, R. (1988) *Anthropometric Standardization Reference Manual*, Human Kinetics Publishers, Champaign.
16.   Astrand, P.-O, Engstrom, L., Eriksson, B.O., Karlberg, P., Nyleer, I., Saltin, B. and Thorén, C. (1963) Girl swimmers. *Acta Paediatrica*, Suppl. 147, pp.43-63.
17.   Lavoie, J.-M. and Monpetit, R.R. (1986) Applied physiology of swimming. Sports Medicine, Vol. 3, pp.165-189.
18.   Toussaint, H.M., Hollander, A.P., deGroot, G., vanIngen Schenau, G.J., Vervoorn, K., Best, H., Meulemans, T. and Schreurs, W. (1988) Measurement of efficiency in swimming man, in *International Series on Sport Sciences: Vol.18. Swimming Science V*, (eds. B.E. Ungerechts, K. Reischle and K. Wilke), Human Kinetics, Champaign, pp. 45-52.

PART SIX

TRAINING ASPECTS

28 A DEVICE FOR QUANTITATIVE MEASUREMENT OF STARTING TIME IN SWIMMING

R. ARELLANO, F.J. MORENO,
M. MARTÍNEZ and A. OÑA
Facultad de las Ciencias de la Actividad Física y el Deporte,
Granada, Spain

Abstract
A device for quantitative measurement of the phases of the starting time was developed using a group of photocells plus one touch-pad attached to a bulkhead. A computer connected by parallel port was used to start and time each phase of the swimmer start (maximun distance: 10-m). Nine male high school swimmers participated in the study. Four different methods were used for covering the 10-m distance: 1) gliding, 2) freestyle kicking, 3) butterfly kicking, and 4) freestyle. The results showed a significant and positive correlation between water phase of the start and total start time. The phases block time 1, block time 2 and flight time showed no correlation. Significant differences between the total time of the four starts used and water time were found. The phases block time 1, block time 2 and flight time didn't show these differences between the four starts. The equipment developed seems useful for training the swimming block-start giving accurate terminal feed-back time. The training of the swimming start has to be primarily oriented to decrease the drag during the water phase.
Keywords: Swimming start technique, swimming start time.

1 Introduction

The time taken from the instant the starting signal is given until a swimmer completes the distance of a race is equal to the time spent starting plus the time spent stroking during each length plus the time spent turning (1) and plus the time spent finishing (2). Each element of the swimming race has a different percentage of contribution of the total time.

An analysis of this type done during international swimming events showed how the importance of time spent starting (the first 10-m) decreased when the race distance increased (2-4), although starting time it is a critical factor in the performance in the shortest events (50-m and 100-m).

Studies of the starting technique in swimming literature divide the swimming start in phases of different duration: hand time, block time, flight time and water time (5-7). These times were obtained in most of the cases using a cinematography method. Only few studies (5,7) used a touchpad mounted on a bulkhead (9 m from the wall) for automatic timing of the total start time during the cinematography study. In this study our aim was to develop a portable system for automatic timing of each phase, able to provide time information to the swimmer after each repetition, as well as evaluate the effectiveness of the system itself.

2 Method

2.1 Subjects
Nine male high school swimmers with more than five years of competitive experience were measured. The mean age was 16.2 years and the means of their anthropometric variables were height =173.3 cm (sd=6.7), body weight = 65,7 kg (sd=11.1), arm span = 180.7 cm (sd=7.9), total body length = 237.6 cm (sd=9.6). The mean of the time of 25-m swimming crawl stroke without block start was 13.7 s (sd=0.85).

2.2 Variables
The starting time was divided into: BT1 (block time 1), the time from the starting signal to the instant the hands leave the block; BT2 (block time 2), the time from the instant the hands leave the block until the feet leave the block at takeoff; FT (flight time), the elapsed time between the instant of takeoff and hand entry; WT (water time), the time from the instant of hand entry until first contact with a bulkhead placed 10 m from the start; ST (start time), the time from the starting signal to the first contact with the bulkhead (Fig. 1).

Fig. 1.   Phases of the swimming start analyzed in this study.

   The start variables were measured for different conditions for each swimmer: a) start and gliding (without propulsion) until touched the bulkhead; b) start and freestyle kicking until touched the bulkhead; c) start and butterfly kicking until touched the bulkhead; and d) start and freestyle swimming until they touched the bulkhead.   A randomized design was used for controlling the order effect.

2.3 Instrumentation
A timing measurement system consisting of three groups of photocells and a touchpad connected to a personal computer by a parallel port was used to record the performance of each trial.   A compiled computer program was used to control the process.   The program was able to record each trial time and produce graphs of phase times for different trials.

3 Results

The means and standard deviations for each phase and type of water time plus the correlation with the starting time are presented in Table 1.   As variables could be influenced by swimmer height , each of the start variables were correlated with ST with subject height partialled out.
   The results showed a high and significant correlation between water time phase and total start time.   This correlation was repeated for each case of water time.   Meanwhile none of the other phases of the start correlated with the start time in any of the water time conditions.

Table 1.   Means, standard deviations and partial correlation of the variables studied, grouped by the type of start analyzed.

Water time condition	Phase	Mean (s)	SD	r
Gliding	BT1	0,592	0,107	-0,104
	BT2	0,312	0,051	0,179
	FT	0,331	0,068	0,002
	WT	4,640	0,818	0,965 p<0,01
	ST	5,875	0,268	
Freestyle kicking	BT1	0,578	0,076	-0,231
	BT2	0,292	0,054	-0,048
	FT	0,337	0,067	-0,503
	WT	3,924	0,752	0,987 p<0,01
	ST	5,131	0,231	
Butterfly kicking	BT1	0,581	0,065	-0,003
	BT2	0,310	0,041	0,119
	FT	0,332	0,043	0,157
	WT	3,774	0,412	0,910 p<0,01
	ST	4,997	0,136	
Freestyle	BT1	0,575	0,045	0,317
	BT2	0,286	0,043	-0,261
	FT	0,351	0,046	-0,245
	WT	3,326	0,460	0,983 p<0,01
	ST	4,539	0,149	

Using the same start time variables duration of each phase under four types of water time (independent variable: IV). The results are summarized in Table 1. Using the ANOVA of repeated measures we tried to find differences on the effect of IV in the time of each phase of the start.

Significant differences were seen between means at the ST and WT phases $F(3,24) = 22,23$ $p<0.01$ and $F(3,24)=23,62$ $p<0,01$, respectively. The Scheffé *post hoc* test showed differences between means in each case. The BT1, BT2 and FT dependent variables did not show significant differences in any case.

4 Discussion

The device developed seems to be a very valuable tool for coaching the start technique. The coach can measure the modifications in duration for each start phase (performed following specific technique instructions) after every repetition. The software shows the evolution for each temporal variable during a instructional period.

Our results showed high correlational values between ST and WT and no correlation with the other phases as in other studies (5, 7); although the start distance was one meter further and the subjects in our experiment used different techniques during water time. Water time accounted for 93%, 97%, 82% and 96% of the variance in the start time.

BT1was longer than BT2 and FT. BT2 and FT were performed with similar times. BT1 includes reaction time and can be different when the swimmer uses variants in start technique like swinging the arms behind or infront of the body. BT2 depends on the angle of take-off used by the swimmer. If the angle is small BT2 will be longer; if the angle is larger BT2 will be shorter.

We found that butterfly kicking was more effective than freestyle kicking in a group of freestylers, an example of the need to further evaluate the use of ondulatory movements during the underwater or swimming phases of the competitive strokes.

The lack of differences between four types of start in phases BT1, BT2 and FT confirmed that these phases were independent of the kind of the start used and that their contribution to the total starting time was very low.

5 Conclusion

On the basis of these findings, it seems appropriate to suggest: 1) the importance of the swimming start in short swimming events, makes it necessary to train this skill in a separate manner using specific equipment to accurately measure the start variables and capable of providing terminal feedback after each repetition; 2) the aim of the swimming start training must be decreasing reaction time, included in BT1 and reducing the water time thanks to a better body position for decreasing the drag during the water entry and during the underwater phase of the start.

6 References

1.   Hay JG. Swimming. (1986) In: Hay JG, ed. *Starting, Stroking & Turning (A Compilation of Research on the Biomechanics of Swimming, The University of Iowa, 1983-86)*. 1st ed. Iowa: Biomechanics Laboratory, Departament of Exercise Science, pp. 1-51.

2. Absaliamov, Timakovoy.(1990) *Aseguramiento Científico de la Competición.* (1 ed.) Moscú: Vneshtorgizdat, pp. 241.

3. Arellano R, Brown P, Cappaert J, Nelson RC. (1994) Analysis of 50-, 100-, and 200-m Freestyle Swimmers at the 1992 Olympic Games. *Journal of Applied Biomechanics*, Vol. 10, pp. 189-199.

4. Absaliamov T, Shircovets E, Lipsky E. (1989) *Analysis of Competitive Activity.(European Swimming Championships)* In: Liga Europea de Natación, :

5. Hay JG, Guimaraes ACS, Grimston SK. (1983) A Quantitive Look at Swimming Biomechanics. In: Hay JG, ed. *Starting, Stroking & Turning (A Compilation of Research on the Biomechanics of Swimming, The University of Iowa, 1983-86).* Iowa: Biomechanics Laboratory, Departament of Exercise Science, pp. 76-82.

6. Miller JA, Hay JG, Wilson BD. (1984) Starting Techniques of Elite Swimmers. *Journal of Sports Science*, Vol. 2, pp. 213-223.

7. Guimaraes A, Hay J. (1984) A Mechanical Analysis of the Grab Starting Technique in Swimming. *International Journal of Sports Biomechanics.* Vol.1, pp. 25-35.

Acknowledgments

This research was supported by "Secretaría General Plan Nacional I+D " (CICYT) - DEP91-0524
Attendance at this Congress was partially supported by the "Federación Española de Natación", the "Comité Olímpico Español" and the "Universidad de Granada".

29 TRAINING CONTENT AND ITS EFFECTS ON PERFORMANCE IN 100 AND 200 M SWIMMERS

I. MUJIKA, T. BUSSO, A. GEYSSANT, J.C. CHATARD
Laboratoire de Physiologie, GIP Exercise,
Faculté de Médecine de Saint-Etienne, France
F. BARALE, L. LACOSTE
Toulouse Olympic Etudiant Club, Toulouse, France

Abstract
The relationships between the mean intensity of a training season, training volume and frequency, and the variations in performance were studied in a group of elite swimmers (N = 18). Additionally, differences between the swimmers who improved their personal record during the season (Fast, n = 8) and those who did not (Slow, n = 10) were searched for. The improvement in performance during the season was significantly correlated with the mean intensity of the training season (r = 0.69, P < 0.01), but not with training volume or frequency. The performance improvement during the season was significantly related to the initial performance level (r = 0.90, P < 0.01). The loss in performance during detraining from the previous season was lower for the group Fast than for the group Slow (6.21 ± 2.30% vs 9.79 ± 2.18%, P < 0.01). The present findings suggest that training intensity is the key factor in the production of a training effect. Factors such as previous detraining and initial performance level could jeopardize success in spite of a good adaptation to training.
Keywords: Blood lactate, detraining, exercise, performance, weight training.

1 Introduction

The training stimulus is usually described as a combination of intensity, volume and frequency [1]. Swimmers have therefore progressively increased their amounts of training up to 10,000 $m \cdot d^{-1}$ in two or three sessions per day [2]. The question of which of the three training components maximizes conditioning and enhances swimming performance remains [3]. As a matter of fact, evaluate training intensity throughout a season requires to code and record each exercise performed by the swimmers during each training session, which is a difficult task for coaches and scientists. Thus, the present study was designed to (i) describe an easy method to estimate the mean intensity of training, volume and frequency of an entire season in a group of elite swimmers; (ii) determine the relationship between these three training components and the variations in performance; (iii) compare the training content of those swimmers who were able to improve their previous season's personal record during the follow-up period (Fast group) with that of the swimmers who did not improve it (Slow group); (iiii) investigate whether performance variations could be related to the performance loss due to the detraining period following the previous swimming season.

2 Methods

2.1 Subjects
The subjects were 18 French national and international level swimmers. Nine of the subjects specialized in the 100 m event, while the other 9 swam the 200 m. Swimmers were divided into two groups, since 8 of them were able to swim $0.65 \pm 0.58\%$ (mean ± SD) faster during the follow-up period (season 1991-92) than they did in 1990-91 (Fast), while the other 10 swam $1.13 \pm 0.96\%$ slower in 1991-92 (Slow). The main characteristics of the two groups of swimmers are shown in Table 1.

Table 1.   Comparison of the two groups of swimmers. Values are means ± SD.

		n	Age (yr)	Height (cm)	Weight (kg)	Competition (yr)
Fast	Female	4	18 ± 1	170 ± 2	57 ± 5	9 ± 4
	Male	4	21 ± 3	187 ± 6	79 ± 14	13 ± 5
	Total	8	20 ± 3	179 ± 10	68 ± 15	11 ± 5
Slow	Female	4	20 ± 1	173 ± 4	60 ± 8	12 ± 1
	Male	6	22 ± 3	184 ± 5	73 ± 5	13 ± 4
	Total	10	21 ± 3	179 ± 7	68 ± 9	13 ± 3

All the differences between groups were statistically non-significant.

2.2 Training
The 1991-92 training program started after detraining from the previous season and was divided into 3 main periods, each one leading to an important competition: wk 14, 29 and 44. The training intensity was measured from blood lactate concentration in the early season after performing 200 m swims at a progressively increased pace. Blood samples were taken from a fingertip during the 1 min rest interval after each 200 m swim. Five training intensity levels were established according to the result of this test: intensity I: swimming speed inferior to 2 mM; intensity II: speed close to 4 mM; intensity III: speed close to 6 mM; intensity IV: highly lactic swimming (10 mM); intensity V:

maximal intensity sprint swimming. All workouts over the season were timed for each swimmer and intensity calculated and categorized according to the five intensity levels. Blood lactate values were measured several times throughout the season, in order to adjust the training intensity level as the lactate response of the swimmers was modified with training. Training volume was the total distance swum, in km, and training frequency the number of half-days of rest. For dryland training, it was empirically considered that 1 h of dryland training was equivalent to 1 km swum at intensity I, 0.5 km at intensity IV and 0.5 km at intensity V.

2.3 Estimation of a stress index scale
A stress index scale was established according to the theoretical blood lactate accumulation levels aimed during the different training sets, as follows: values 2, 4, 6 and 10 mM corresponded to the intensity levels I, II, III and IV, respectively. The corresponding value for intensity V was estimated as 16. These values were then divided by two, in order to make them more manageable. Thus, the index scale was 1, 2, 3, 5, 8, to be multiplied by the distance swum at each intensity level.

2.4 Mean intensity of the training season (MITS)
To estimate the value of the entire season's mean intensity of training for each swimmer, the total distance swum at intensities I, II, III, IV, and V were multiplied by the stress indexes 1, 2, 3, 5 and 8, respectively, and the calculated equivalents of dryland training were added to the computation. Then, the MITS value was computed as;
$(1 \text{ kmI} + 2 \text{ kmII} + 3 \text{ kmIII} + 5 \text{ kmIV} + 8 \text{ kmV} + \text{dryland equivalent}) / \text{volume}$

2.5 Performance
Each swimmer's best performance of the season was compared with the initial one, and the difference was expressed as the percentage of change. It was observed that each swimmer's first performance of the season was completed with an evident lack of motivation. Therefore, this first performance was discounted and the second one was chosen to determine the initial performance level of each swimmer.

2.6 Statistical analysis
Means and standard deviations were calculated for all the variables. Correlations between the training variables and the variation in performance were calculated from linear regression. Comparisons between the groups Fast and Slow were treated with a Student t - test for unpaired samples. The 0.05 level of significance was adopted.

3 Results

3.1 Training
For the whole group of swimmers, the mean ± SD training volume was 1126 ± 222 km (range from 749 to 1475), the training frequency 316 ± 44 half days of rest (range from 264 to 370), the dryland training 1108 ± 828 min (range from 0 to 2415). The mean ± SD percentages of the total distance covered at each intensity were 77.4 ± 3.1; 11.2 ± 2.7; 6.6 ± 0.9; 3.7 ± 0.2 and 1.0 ± 0.2 for intensity I, II, III, IV and V, respectively. The mean intensity of the training season (MITS) was calculated to correspond to 1.53 ± 0.06 arbitrary units (range 1.42 - 1.64).

3.2 Training - Performance relationship
For the 18 swimmers, MITS was related to the improvement in performance throughout the season (r = 0.69; P < 0.01; Fig. 1A). On the other hand, no significant correlation was found between the improvement in performance and the training volume or the training frequency. Improvements were related to the initial performance of the season: the lower the decline in performance from the previous season, the smaller the improvement during the follow-up period (r = 0.90; P < 0.01).

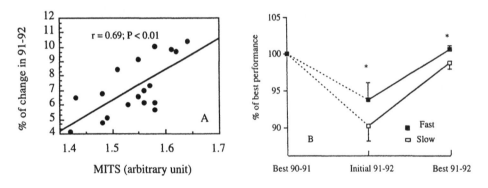

Fig. 1. Relationship between the improvement in performance throughout the follow-up period (91-92) and the mean intensity of training during the season (A); variations between the best performance of the season 90-91 and the initial performance of the follow-up period (91-92), and between the latter and the best of the same season (B). The values are expressed as a percentage of the best performance achieved in 1990-91. * denotes a significant difference between the two groups (P < 0.01).

3.3 Fast and Slow group comparison
No significant difference existed in the MITS, training volume, frequency or dryland training between groups (Table 2). However, a significant difference (P < 0.01) was

found in the amount of loss between the best performance of the previous season and the initial performance of 1991-92. Indeed, while the group Slow had a loss in performance of 9.79 ± 2.18%, the group Fast decreased only by 6.21 ± 2.30% (Fig. 1B). The amount of improvement in performance throughout the season 1991-92 was not significantly different for the groups Fast and Slow, even though the mean values were slightly higher for the latter: 6.65 ± 1.00% vs 7.66 ± 1.95%.

Table 2.   Comparison of the total values of all the quantified training variables during the season 1991-92. All the variables are measured in km, except for Frequency in 1/2 days of rest, Weight training in min and MITS in arbitrary units.

Variable	Fast		Slow	
	Mean	SD	Mean	SD
Frequency	305.8	41.8	345.8	57.3
Volume	1151.3	189.3	1055.1	250.3
Intensity I	885.5	138.5	813.9	169.7
Intensity II	131.9	41.9	120.4	56.3
Intensity III	76.8	19.7	69.7	22.7
Intensity IV	42.6	8.3	38.5	8.3
Intensity V	11.2	2.2	10.8	2.1
Weight Training	901.3	925.5	1273.0	749.7
MITS	1.52	0.07	1.56	0.06

All the differences between groups were non-significant.

4 Discussion

For the present group of elite swimmers, a positive correlation was observed between the improvement in performance achieved during the season and the estimated mean intensity of their training program. Thus, the intensity of the training bout seems to be the key factor in producing the desired training effect [4]. It is questionable, however, whether this possibility could be extended to swimmers of longer distances (400 to 1500 m), since training volume and frequency could be much more important for those swimmers. Different experimental results suggest that high intensity training should be included in the programs for sprinters. When an exercise lasts between 1 and 2 min, the relative part of anaerobic energy release varies between 35 and 60% [5]. Four hundred and 800 m runners have an anaerobic capacity 30% higher than endurance trained athletes or sedentary subjects [6]. The same authors have shown that a 6-wk training period, including intensive exercises produced a gain of 10% in anaerobic capacity, which should lead to a reduction of several seconds in any event lasting 1 to 3 min [6].

The influence of training frequency and volume on performance, found for untrained subjects previously [1, 4], was not observed in the present highly trained swimmers. This difference may indicate the possible existence of a training stimulus threshold, beyond which intensity would be the main factor in the production of a training effect. Indeed, it has been shown that doubling the training volume of a group of collegiate swimmers during 6 weeks did not result in higher aerobic or anaerobic capacities. Furthermore, the swimmers did not improve their swimming power but decreased their maximal sprinting velocity during that period [3]. Another study has shown that in spite of a reduction in the training volume from an average of 8741 m·d⁻¹ to 4517 m·d⁻¹ over two competitive seasons, $\dot{V}O_{2max}$ or blood lactate after a standard 183 m swim did not change, while swimming power and performance were significantly improved [7]. It might be erroneously concluded that low intensity training is not useful for short distance swimmers. A high volume of low intensity training could improve the recovery process and make high intensity training easier to tolerate [4], and could also improve the gliding ability, reducing the energy cost of swimming [8, 9].

The individual response to a training regime seems to depend on the level of fitness of a subject [1, 4]. In the present study, a highly significant correlation was observed between the initial level of performance of the season and the improvement in performance during the season. Furthermore, the percentage loss in performance during the period separating the personal record of 1990-91 and the beginning of the season 1991-92 was significantly different for the groups Fast and Slow. This fact seems to be closely related with the concept of detraining, since most of the swimmers were at their highest level at the end of the previous season, immediately before the summer break. Since these negative effects appear to be much less important when the swimmers continue to train at a minimum level of 30% of the previous training effort [10], the present swimmers would have perhaps benefited more from a reduced training at the end of the season rather than from inactivity.

In summary, the results of the study showed that training intensity, rather than training volume or frequency, was the key factor in the production of a training effect. Also, it was concluded that previous detraining and the level of performance at the beginning of the season could jeopardize athletic success in spite of a good adaptation to training.

5 References

1. Wenger, H.A. and Bell, G.J. (1986) The interactions of intensity, frequency and duration of exercise training in altering cardiorespiratory fitness. *Sports Medicine*, Vol. No. 3, pp. 346-356.
2. Costill, D.L. (1985) Practical problems in exercise physiology research. *Research Quarterly for Exercise and Sport*, Vol. No. 56, pp. 378-384.
3. Costill, D.L., Thomas, R., Robergs, R.A, Pascoe, D., Lambert, C., Barr, S., and Fink, W.J. (1991) Adaptations to swimming training: influence of training volume. *Medicine and Science in Sports and Exercise*, Vol. No. 23, pp. 371-377.

4.   Shepard, R. (1968) Intensity, duration and frequency of exercise as determinants of the response to a training regime. *Internationale Zeitschrift fur Angewante Physiologie,* Vol. No. 26, pp. 272-278.

5.   Medbø, J.I. and Tabata I. (1989) Relative importance of aerobic and anaerobic energy release during short-lasting exhausting bicycle exercise. *Journal of Applied Physiology,* Vol. No. 67, pp. 1881-1886.

6.   Medbø, J.I., and Burgers S. (1990) Effect of training on the anaerobic capacity. *Medicine and Science in Sports and Exercise,* Vol. No. 22, pp. 501-507.

7.   Costill, D.L., Fink, W.J., Hargreaves, M., King, D.S., Thomas, R., Fielding R. (1985) Metabolic characteristics of skeletal muscle during detraining from competitive swimming. *Medicine and Science in Sports and Exercise,* Vol. No. 17, pp. 339-343.

8.   Sharp, R.L. (1993) Prescribing and evaluating interval training sets in swimming: a proposed model. *Journal of Swimming Research,* Vol. No. 9, pp. 36-40.

9.   Chatard, J.C., Lavoie, J.M. and Lacour J.R. (1990) Analysis of determinants of swimming economy in front crawl. *European Journal of Applied Physiology,* Vol. No. 61, pp. 88-92.

10.   Neufer, P.D., Costill, D.L., Fielding, R.A., Flynn, M.G., Kirwan J.P. (1987) Effect of reduced training on muscular strength and endurance in competitive swimmers. *Medicine and Science in Sports and Exercise,* Vol. No. 19, pp. 486-490.

30 PHYSIOLOGICAL EVALUATION OF THE 400 M FREESTYLE RACE

T. NOMURA
Kyoto Institute of Technology, Kyoto, Japan
K. WAKAYOSHI
Nara University of Education, Nara, Japan
M. MIYASHITA and Y. MUTOH
The University of Tokyo, Tokyo, Japan

Abstract
The purpose of this study was to physiologically evaluate performance on a 400 m freestyle race with consideration of the aerobic-anaerobic relation to swimming velocity. The subjects were 21 male and 26 female swimmers who participated at the 1993 Pan Pacific Swimming Championships in Kobe, Japan. The velocity was evaluated by using the aerobic/anaerobic velocity model. This model included aerobic velocity and fatigue effect. The third root of exponential function for course of time was used as a parameter of aerobic velocity. Further, a linear function for course of time was applied to a parameter of fatigue effect. During the race, the aerobic power contributed $57.98 \pm 1.94\%$ of the total energy expenditure for males and $56.35 \pm 3.14\%$ for females. Though anaerobic energy contributed primarily only during the first stage of race, there was no significant correlation between the anaerobic velocity during this phase and the average velocity of the entire race. It was noteworthy that a high relation existed between aerobic velocity and total velocity during the mid stage portion of the race. A correlation for male ($r = 0.454$, $p < 0.01$) between the average velocity of the entire race and the anaerobic velocity during the last stage was contrasted with the value for female ($r = -0.130$, NS.).
Keywords: Physiological evaluation, 400m freestyle, race, velocity, aerobic, anaerobic.

1 Introduction

In 400m freestyle competitive swimming, it is necessary to pace oneself. Both aerobic and anaerobic processes contribute to the energy release in this event [1,2,3]. Swimming velocity influences the rate of energy production and fatigue. Many models concerning oxygen uptake kinetics during exercise that are based on exponential function have been developed from experimental data [4,5,6]. Lactate concentration has a significant correlation with swimming velocity [7]. Great increases in swimming performances have followed the results of such findings. However, it is impossible to obtain physiological data during the race. Therefore, the purpose of this study was physiologically evaluate performance on a 400m freestyle race with consideration of the aerobic-anaerobic relation to swimming velocity.

2 Methods

2.1 Sampling method
The subjects were 21 male and 26 female swimmers who participated at the 1993 Pan Pacific Swimming Championships in Kobe, Japan [8].

Eight split times were taken from the official electric timer. Passing time 10m from the start, 5m before turns (turn-in), 7.5m after turns (turn-out), and 5m before the goal were read from a video timer superimposed upon video images of the race.

2.2 Adjustment of split time
The effects of the start and finish were removed from these split times. The start time was replaced with an average time of turn-out, and first swimming time was adjusted to the time during 37.5m. The finish time was replaced with an average time of turn-in. Each split time was calculated as that equaling turn-out time plus Stroke time plus turn-in time.

2.3 Evaluation method
Oxygen uptake kinetics is approximated as an exponential function of the course of time [9,10]. O2 uptake subtracted from O2 demand is O2 debt [11,12]. Oxygen uptake is a parameter of aerobic energy production capability. On the other hand, oxygen debt is a parameter of anaerobic energy production capability. Therefore, a single-exponential function was chosen as a basic model on production kinetics of aerobic energy (Eq.1). Moreover, a time constant of 40 second for this equation was chosen based upon results from previous studies [10,13,14].

$$\text{Aerobic energy consumption} \ \spadesuit \ (1-e^{-t/\tau}) \tag{1}$$

where t shows the course of time, and τ indicates time constant (40sec.).

The power output is reflected by the velocity cubed. This is because propulsion varies in proportion as the velocity squared, and the power varies in proportion as the propulsion is multiplied by the velocity [15]. Therefore, the aerobic velocity is described as the third root of aerobic energy.

However, during high intensity exercise, the single-exponential function can not explain pure oxygen uptake kinetics [16,17]. The aerobic power production is involved in the anaerobic power production. The anaerobic power production brings about increases in some metabolic by-products associates with fatigue [18]. Lactate, which is one of those metabolic by-products, concentrates linearly to the time course during high intensity exercise[19,20]. The accumulation of fatigue limits the aerobic power output [13].

On the supposition that a constant anaerobic power was yielded (C_{an}), the fatigue effect was described as Eq.2:

$$\text{Fatigue effect} = a\,t + b \tag{2}$$

Here, "a" and "b" were estimated from velocities of the middle stage of race that was measured between 4th and 6th split (150m to 300m), because velocity changes during this stage slightly. Further, the third root of aerobic power reaches 98% of steady state until 120 sec in this exponential model. The "a" indicates the intensity of fatigue effect. The "b" shows a state without any fatigue.

Accordingly, the basic aerobic velocity (B_{aer}) was regressed as follows:

$$B_{aer} = \sqrt[3]{(1-e^{-t/40}) \cdot (at + b) - C_{an}} \tag{3}$$

Though C_{an} is an unknown quantity, a range of it is larger than zero and smaller than third root term of Eq.3 at the first split. Moreover, O2 uptake kinetics has a time delay of a couple of seconds at onset of exercise [6]. Hence, the C_{an} was supposed as half

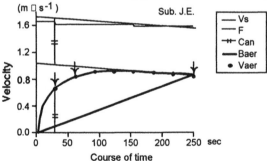

Vs; Swimming velocity = 50 m · (Turn-out time+ Stroke time + Turn-in time)$^{-1}$.
F; Effect of fatigue that was regressed from *Vs* between 150m to 300m.
Can; Supposed constant anaerobic velocity. Baer; Basic aerobic velocity.
Vaer; Aerobic velocity that was considered anaerobic velocity variation.
Baer curve was transformed to Vaer in the direction of arrow.

Fig. 1. Simplified explanation of relation velocities.

of third root term of Eq.3 at the first split.

$$C_{an} = 0.5 \cdot \sqrt[3]{(1-e^{-t/40})} \cdot (at_1 + b) \tag{4}$$

on condition that is t_1 = time of the first split.

Basic Anaerobic velocity (B_{an}) in the basic model was obtained as the swimming velocity minus B_{aer}. However, the real production of anaerobic power shows some variation [21]. The adjusted fatigue effect was calculated from Ban, Can and the slope of Eq.2.

$$a'_n = a \cdot B_{an} / C_{an} \tag{5}$$

For keeping continuous aerobic velocities, the constant "b" was adjusted using a data point that is the fourth split (150 to 200m).

$$
\begin{aligned}
b'_n &= (a - a'_n) \cdot t_n + b & (n = 4) \\
b'_n &= (a'_n - a'_{n+1}) \cdot t_n + b'_{n+1} & (n < 4) \\
b'_n &= (a'_{n-1} - a'_n) \cdot t_n + b'_{n-1} & (n > 4)
\end{aligned}
\tag{6}
$$

Hence, the aerobic (V_{aer}) and anaerobic (V_{an}) velocity was calculated as follow:

$$
\begin{aligned}
V_{aer} &= \sqrt[3]{(1-e^{-t/40})} \cdot (a't + b') - C_{an} \\
V_{an} &= V_s - V_{aer}
\end{aligned}
\tag{7}
$$

Aerobic power contributions were calculated as $V_{aer}^3 / (V_{aer}^3 + V_{an}^3) \cdot 100$.
Fig. 1 shows a simplified explanation of relation velocities.

3 Results

3.1 Aerobic / anaerobic

Table 1 shows calculated swimming velocities and the aerobic power contribution during 400m race. For male swimmers, the aerobic power contribution to each point was as follows; $19.7 \pm 1.8\%$ at 50 m, $55.6 \pm 2.5\%$ at 100 m, 68.3 - 73.2% during 150

Table 1. Swimming velocity and Contribution of aerobic power

Split	Distance m	Male (n=21) Swim velosity m⊡sec	Cont. of aero %	Female (n=26) Swim velosity m⊡sec	Cont. of aer %
1	50	1.742 ± 0.026	19.69± 1.78	1.609 ± 0.031	21.12± 2.21
2	100	1.671 ± 0.022	55.57± 2.47	1.554 ± 0.030	54.87± 2.48
3	150	1.662 ± 0.031	68.33± 1.42	1.533 ± 0.035	67.95± 1.19
4	200	1.650 ± 0.033	73.15± 1.46	1.523 ± 0.036	71.34± 2.30
5	250	1.654 ± 0.033	73.03± 2.73	1.524 ± 0.041	70.71± 2.51
6	300	1.645 ± 0.032	72.77± 2.49	1.510 ± 0.041	70.24± 3.95
7	350	1.654 ± 0.034	69.23± 5.84	1.516 ± 0.044	66.02± 7.28
8	400	1.686 ± 0.052	62.19± 7.36	1.530 ± 0.045	59.58±11.53

Swimming velocity = 50 m · (Turn-out time+ Stroke time + Turn-in time)$^{-1}$
Cont. of aero = (aerobic velocity)^3 · {(aerobic velocity)^3+(anaerobic velocity)^3}$^{-1}$ · 100

to 350 m, and 62.19 ± 7.4% at 400 m. When the aerobic power integrated with respect to the course of time, the aerobic energy contributed 57.98 ± 1.94% to the total energy output for horizontal direction. For female swimmers, the aerobic power contribution showed a similar tendency to that of male swimmers. On the whole, the aerobic energy contributed 56.35 ± 3.14% to the total energy output for horizontal direction.

3.2 Relation between total velocity and aerobic/anaerobic velocity

The correlation between the total velocity and aerobic/anaerobic velocities are shown for Fig.2. For male swimmers, the coefficients of correlation between total velocity and aerobic velocity during 1st to 6th split were significant (0.72 to 0.97, $p<0.01$). However, the significant correlation between the average velocity of the entire race and anaerobic velocities were obtained only in the 3rd 4th 6th and 8th split. For female swimmers, The correlation between total velocity and aerobic velocities during each split were all significant. A significant correlation between the average velocity of entire race and anaerobic velocities was obtained only during the 2nd to 6th split. In 8th split, this correlation for male ($r = 0.454$, $p <0.01$) was contrast with the value for female ($r = -0.130$, NS.).

4 Discussion

Contribution of aerobic energy in the 400 m freestyle race in this study was smaller than that found by others [22]. One possible explanation was that swimmers in this study did not keep an even pace during the first stage and final stage of the race. Further, total mechanical power involves not only propelling power but also rotational power of body segments [23]. Stroke frequency is strongly dependent on swimming

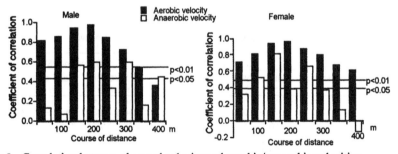

Fig.2. Correlation between the total velocity and aerobic/anaerobic velocities

velocity [24]. Some additional power is generally considered to be necessary to change pace during swimming. As the energy contribution estimation value was close to other literature values [2,25], it seems that this evaluation method has validity.

Though anaerobic power contributed mainly during the first stage of the race, there was no significant correlation between the anaerobic velocity during this phase and the average velocity of the entire race. Accordingly, it is necessary for a male swimmer to save anaerobic power during the first stage and to concentrate it after 300 m. On the other hand, female swimmers had a more constant relation between aerobic velocity and the average velocity of entire race. Therefore, emphasis for the female swimmer should be to swim fast with low fatigue during the mid portion of the race. Maximal swimming velocity in the 400 m event significantly correlated with the stroke technique on the energy cost [3,26].

Unlike the results of the males, the females had no significant correlation between the average velocity of entire race and anaerobic velocity during the last stage of the race. Females had a tendency to use anaerobic power during mid portion of the race. It seems that it is difficult to concentrate anaerobic power for females because anaerobic capacity closely follows improvement in muscle mass [27].

5 Conclusions

These data suggest that the importance of stroke technique in conserving energy during first phase of a 400 m freestyle race. This was because anaerobic power was the main contributor during the first phase of the race. It is noteworthy that a high relation existed between aerobic velocity and total velocity during mid phase. Therefore, it is necessary to not only engage in high intensity training but also aerobic training in preparation for the 400 m freestyle race.

6 References

1. Troup, J.P., Hollander, A.P., Bone, M., Trappe, S. and Barzdukas, A.P. (1992) Performance related differences in the anaerobic contribution of competitive freestyle swimmers, In *Biomechanics and medicine in swimming Swimming science VI*, (ed. D.MacLaren, T.Reilly, and A.Lees), E & FN Spon, London, pp. 271-7.

2. Maglischo, E.W. (1993) *Swimming even faster. Chapter1: E nergy metabolism and swimming performance*, Mayfield Publishing Co., Mountain View, CA, pp.3-22.

3. Ribeiro, J.P., Cadavid, E., Baena, J., Monsalvete, E., Barna, A. and DeRose, E.H. (1990) Metabolic predictors of middle-distance swimming performance. *Bri.J.Sports Medicine* , Vol. 24, No. 3. pp.196-200.

4.   Di Prampero, P.E., Mahler, P.B., Giezendanner, D. and Cerretelli, P. (1989) Effects of priming exercise on VO2 kinetics and O2 deficit at the onset of stepping and cycling. *J.Appl. Physiol.*, Vol. 66, No. 5. pp. 2023-31.

5.   Whipp, B.J., Ward, S.A., Lamarra, N., Davis, J.A. and Wasserman, K. (1982) Parameters of ventilatory and gas exchange dynamics during exercise. *J. Appl.Physiol.* , Vol.52, No.6. pp.1506-13.

6.   Hughson, R.L. and Morrissey, M. (1982) Delayed kinetics of respiratory gas exchange in the transition form prior exercise. *J. Appl.Physiol.* , Vol. 52, No. 4. pp.921-9.

7.   Olbrecht, J., Madsen, Ø., Mader, A., Liesen, H. and Hollmann, W. (1985) Relationship between swimming velocity and lactic concentration during continuous and intermittent   training exercises. *Int.j.sports medicine* , Vol. 6, No. 2. pp.74-7.

8.   Japan Amateur Swimming Federation Medical and Scientific Committee (1993) *Analysis of swimming events at the 1993 Pan Pacific Swimming Championships*, Japan Amateur Swimming Federation, Tokyo, pp.1-109.

9.   Margaria, R., Mangili, F., Cuttica, F. and Cerretelli, P. (1965) The kinetics of the oxygen consumption at the onset of muscular exercise in man. *Ergonomics*, Vol. 8, pp.49-54.

10.   Armon, Y., Cooper, D.M., Flores, R., Zanconato, S. and Barstow, T.J. (1991) Oxygen uptake dynamics during high-intensity exercise in children and adults. *J.Appl.Physiol.*, Vol.70, No. 2. pp.841-8 .

11.   Di Prampero, P.E., Davies, C.T.M., Cerretelli, P. and Margaria, R. (1970) An analysis of O2 debt contracted in submaximal exercise. *J.Appl.Physiol.*, Vol.29, No.5. pp.547-51.

12.   Johnson, A.T. (1991) *Biomechanics and exercise physiology. Chapter 1: Exercise limitations*,   John Wiley & Sons, Inc., New York,NY, pp.1-30.

13.   Hagberg, J.M., Nagle, F.J. and Carlson, J.L. (1978) Transient O2 uptake response at the onset of exercise. *J.AppliPhysiol.*, Vol. 44, No.1. pp.90-2.

14.   Casaburi, R., Barstow, T.J., Robinson, T. and Wasserman, K. (1989) Influence of work rate   on ventilatory and gas exchange kinetics. *J.Appli.Physiol.*, Vol. 67, No. 2. pp. 547-55.

15.   Toussaint, H.M., Hollander, A.P., deGroot, G., vanIngenSchenau, G.J., Vervoorn, K., deBest, H., Meulemans, T. and Schreurs, W. (1988) Measurement of efficiency in swimming man, In *Swimming science V*, (ed. B.E.Ungerechts, K.Wilke, and K.Reischle), Human   Kinetics Pub., Champaign, IL, pp.45-52.

16.   Barstow, T.J., Casaburi, R. and Wasserman, K. (1993) O2 uptake kinetics and the O2 deficit as related to exercise intensity and blood lactate. *J.Appl.Physiol.*, Vol.75, No.2. pp.755-62.

17.   Linnarsson, D. (1974) Dynamics of pulmonary gas exchange and heart rate change at start and end of exercise. *Acta Physiol. Scand.*, Suppl.415, pp.1-68.

18. Roberts, D. and Smith,D.J. (1989) Biochemical aspects of peripheral muscle fatigue. *Sports Medicine*, Vol.7, pp.125-38.
19. Gollnick, P.D. and Hermansen, L. (1973) Biochemical adaptations to exercise: anaerobic metabolism. In *Exercise and Sport Sciences Reviews*, (ed. Wilmore) Vol.1, Academic Press, New York, pp.1-43.
20. Mader, A., Heck, H. and Hollman, W. (1983) A computer simulation model of energy output in relation to metabolic rate and internal environment, *Biochemistry of Exercise*, (ed. H.G. Knuttgen, J.A.Vogel and J.Poortmans), Human Kinetics Pub., Champaign, pp.239-51.
21. Barzdukas,A., Franciosi,P., Trappe,S., Letner,C. and Troup,J.P. (1992) Adaptations to interval training at common intensities and different work : rest ratios, *Biomechanics and medicine in swimming Swimming science VI* , (ed. D. MacLaren, T.Reilly and A.Lees), E&FN Spon, London, pp.359-64.
22. Troup, J.D. (1990) Energy contributions of competitive freestyle events, IN *International Center for Aquatic Research annual: studies by the International Center for Aquatic Research 1989-90*, United States Swimming Press, Colorado Springs, CO, pp.13-9.
23. Toussaint, H.M. (1992) Performance determining factors in front crawl swimming, IN *Biomechanics and medicine in swimming Swimming science VI*, (ed. D.MacLaren, T. Reilly and A. Lees), E&FN Spon, London, pp.13-32.
24. Keskinen, K.L. and Komi, P.V. (1988) Interaction between aerobic/anaerobic loading and biomechanical performance in freestyle swimming, IN *Swimming science V*, (ed. B.E. Ungerechts, K.Wilke and K.Reischle), Human Kinetics Pub., Champaign, IL, pp.285-93.
25. Saltin, B. (1975) *Intermittent Exercise: Its physiology and practical application*, Ball St.U., Muncie, IN, pp.1-28.
26. Costill, D.L., Kovaleski, J., Porter, D., Kirwan, J., Fielding, R. and King, D. (1985) Energy expenditure during front crawl swimming: predicting success in middle-distance events. *Int.J.Sports Medicine*, Vol.6, No.5. pp.266-70.
27. Takahashi, S., Bone, M., Spry, S., Trappe, S. and Troup, J.P. (1992) Differences in the anaerobic power of age group swimmers, IN *Biomechanics and medicine in swimming Swimming science VI*, E & FN Spon, London, (ed. D.MacLaren, T. Reilly and A. Lees), pp.289-94.

31 EFFECTS OF POOL LENGTH ON BIOMECHANICAL PERFORMANCE IN FRONT CRAWL SWIMMING

K.L. KESKINEN, O.P. KESKINEN and A. MERO
Aquatics Research Laboratory
Department of Biology of Physical Activity
University of Jyväskylä, Finland

Abstract

Various external conditions in and outside the water have been shown to affect the performances while swimming. This study aimed to investigate effects of pool length in two series of exercises in both 25-m and 50-m pools. This was done by examining the maximum turning speed to observe the effects of turning skill on the results obtained in the two training conditions. The biomechanical performances were evaluated by the stroke rate, stroke length and mean velocity in five 200-m swims. Turning benefit was measured by underwater filming as a percentage speed gain during turning in comparison with normal all-out swimming. Metabolic effects were examined by the measument of blood lactate concentration and heart rate. The results demonstrated considerable effects of turning skill on the observed differences between the two testing conditions. Extra turns could be seen to allow longer stroke length throughout the short course swims as compared to long course. Elite swimmers could gain more advantage from the turns than their less-good counterparts.
Keywords: Front Crawl, Pool Length, Stroke Length, Stroke Rate

1 Introduction

Competitive swimming results have been ranked separately in short and long course races due to significant differences in performance times. Faster times in short course swimming as compared to long course have been considered mainly because of extra turns. Wirtz et. al. [1] compared stroke length (SL), stroke rate (SR) and mean velocity (v) of highly skilled swimmers having raced both in a 25-m and 50-m pool. They concluded that the swimmers, especially men, could gain advantage from the 25-m pool due to increased speed immediately after the turns. However, there is a lack of research concerning both the biomechanic and metabolic effects [2] of pool length in swimming training. This study, therefore, aimed to evaluate the SR, SL, and v during Aerobic/Anaerobic loading between 25-m and 50-m pools. And, also, this study aimed to examine the maximum turning speed in order to find out the effects of turning skill on the results obtained in the two training conditions.

2 Methods

The subjects were eleven male athletes; three swimmers, six tri-athlonists, and two fin-swimmers. Their physical and performance characteristics are shown in table 1. The subjects performed two training sessions in randomised order with two days of recovery in-between. The exercises consisted of five 200-m front crawl swims in both 25-m and 50-m pool. Starting speed was set according to a 200-m test swim (Time$_{200}$ in table 1), by adding 50 s to the test time. Thereafter, the speed was increased by 10 s in each of the successive 200-m swims. The last swim was performed with maximum effort independent from the previous swims. The swimming speed was adjusted with successive lights underwater and controlled by hand held watches. The two training sessions were performed with equal procedure and times per swim by pre-programming the successive light device according to the test swim. The warm-up procedure included stretching exercises, 15 min of easy swimming, and a set of two or three 200-m swims at the starting velocity of the test exercise.

Table 1. Physical and Performance Characteristics of the subjects.

	Age (y)	Stature (cm)	Mass (kg)	V$_{max}$ (m$*$s^{-1})	Time$_{200}$ (s)	F$_{swim}$ (kg)	CMJ (cm)
Mean	24.7	178.8	73.9	1.55	147.9	13.01	37.2
S.D.	5.0	6.7	6.6	0.13	12.8	2.31	4.6

Blood samples (25 μl) were taken from hyperemisized ear lobes before and after each swim, and 1, 3 and 5 min after the last 200-m swim to analyse blood lactate (BLa) concentration [3]. Time for each swim and for each 50-m and 25-m lap were registered by hand held watches to calculate v (m$*$s^{-1}), correspondingly. Time for ten and five strokes for the 50-m and 25-m pools, in each of the pool lengths during the 200-m swims, were measured to calculate SR (cycles$*$s^{-1}). SL (m$*$cycle^{-1}) was obtained dividing v by SR. Turning skill was measured by underwater filming. Percentage difference between maximum swimming speed just before the flip turn and the turning itself was considered as an index of turning benefit (TB). Maximum swimming force (F$_{swim}$ in table 1) was measured in tethered swimming [4]. The rise of the the center of gravity in centimeters (CMJ in table 1) was evaluated on a contact mat according to the flight time in counter movement vertical jump [5].

The individual graphs for BLa and HR in the function of v, percentage v from the test maximum (v$_R$), and v at metabolic thresholds (v$_T$) were used to average the individual curves of the whole sample. The points of aerobic (AerT) and anaerobic thresholds (AT) were estimated according to the BLa versus v relationship. Means and standard deviations were calculated for the parameters. Correlation coefficients were computed between the variables, and Student t-test for paired observations were used to test the statistical significance (p<0.05) of differences.

3 Results

The two test series demonstrated similar progression of speed throughout the testing, average velocities being closely comparable. The 25-m swims were only slightly faster than 50-m swims. Maximum swims, however, were performed significantly faster (4.8 %) in the 25-m pool. The averaged BLa versus v -curves showed significantly higher BLa values for the 50-m pool as compared to 25-m pool at each v-level throughout the test, and the difference became more pronounced in the latter part of the exercise. A non-significant difference was found in resting and initial levels of BLa. HR values were similar only at maximum speeds.

SL versus v -curves demonstrated statistically significant differences of 1.8 - 8.2 % throughout the tests. When the comparisons were made according to SL versus v (fig.1) in percentage from the test maximum (v_R), the two curves were significantly different by 1.7 - 6.2 %. However, no significant differences could be observed in SR versus v comparisons between the 25- and 50-m pools, neither in terms of absolute v nor v_R (fig. 2).

When the comparisons were made according to v in metabolic thresholds (v_T) it was shown that the swimmers could keep control over SL at a higher speed in the 25-m pool swims as compared to the 50-m pool swims. The collapse point in SL versus v_T-curve, however, was found at the anaerobic threshold in both of the cases (fig. 3). No difference was found in SR versus v_T comparisons. The TB during short maximum swims around the turning wall of the swimming pool averaged 8.2 %, ranging between 15.5% and 4.4%. F_{swim} during tethered swimming (table 1) was found to correlate positively (r=0.786; p<0.01) with the turning velocity and consequently elite swimmers were observed to gain more advantage from the turns than their less-good counterparts.

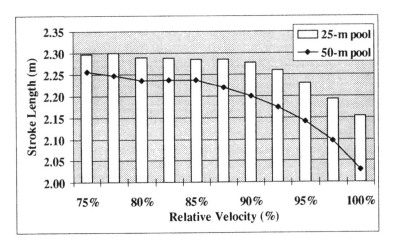

Fig. 1. Stroke Length versus Mean Velocity in relative scale.

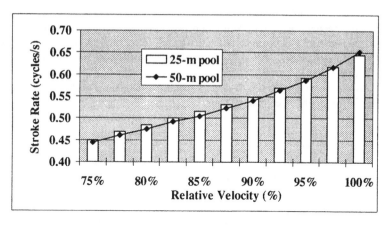

Fig. 2. Stroke Rate versus Mean Velocity in relative scale.

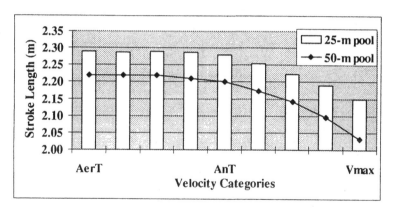

Fig. 3. Stroke Length versus Velocity in Relation to Metabolic Thresholds.

4 Discussion

The major findings of the study demonstrated considerable effects of pool length on both biomechanical performance and metabolic factors. A minor reduction in SR and a minor increase in v during short course swimming, in conjunction with the turns, resulted in a significant increase in SL. On the other hand, Bla levels as well as HR were noted to be significantly higher in 50-m pool swims as compared with 25-m pool swims at each consequtive velocity, except for HR in maximum speeds. Thus it seems that even a short break during stroking may lead to a lengthening of SL and hence to a better performance in the entire swims.

Each turn enabled short breaks (i.e. 4-6 s) during stroking, and in a 200-m swim there were four extra turns to be used for sudden relief for the arm and upper body musculature. Consequently, it became more easy to swim in the 25-m pool as compared to the 50-m pool. The findings of Hultmann & al. [6] may support this suggestion as if even a few seconds break may restore a part of the high energy phosphagens which have been consumed during physical activity. Thereafter, in the present situation, these stores could be used again during the early part of the subsequent pool lengths during the five 200-m swims [7].

While the training in the 25-m pool seems less strenuous than in 50-m pool it must be taken into account when making plans for training. Swimmers that usually train in short course should also train in the 50-m pools in order to get accustomed to official and, as demonstrated by the present data, to more strenuous competitive circumstances. On the other hand, training in the 25-m pool may help swimmers to develop their arm stroke patterns while the short course swimming allows a better swimming velocity with a more efficient stroking as seen from the longer SL during 25-m pool swimming.

Effects of pool length should also be taken into account when performing exercise testing for the aquatic athletes. The present data suggest that in order to fully understand the conditioning process taking place during continuous swimming training the physiological testing should be performed in a situation that would be similar to those where the swimmers execute their daily training practice.

It was concluded that the turning skill was the major factor to determine the observed differences between the two testing conditions. The extra turns throughout the short course training could be seen to allow longer SL as compared with long course swims.

5 References

Wirtz, W., Wilke, K. and Zimmermann, F. (1992) Velocity, distance per stroke and stroke frequency of highly skilled swimmers in 50-m freestyle sprint in a 50 and 25-m pool. In (eds D. MacLaren, T. Reilly and A. Lees) Biomechanics and Medicine in Swimming; Swimming Science VI. E & FN SPON, Chapman & Hall, London, p. 131-134.

Keskinen, O.P., Keskinen, K.L. and Mero A. (1994) Effect of Pool Length in Exercise Testing of Swimmers. International Journal of Sports Medicine. (submitted)

Böhringer-Mannheim: Test-Fibel. (1979) Enzymatische Bestimmung von Lactat im Plasma, Blut und Liquor [Enzymatic Determination of Lactate in plasma, blood and fluids]. Mannheim.

Keskinen, K.L., Tilli, L.J. and Komi, P.V. (1989) Maximum Velocity Swimming: Interrelationships of Stroking Characteristics, Force Production, and Anthropometric Variables. Scandinavian Journal of Sports Sciences, 11 (2), 87-92.

Komi, P.V. and Bosco, C. (1978) Utilization of Stored Elastic Energy in Men and Women. Medicine and Science in Sports, 10, 261-265.

Hultman, E., Bergström, J. and McLennan Andersson, N. (1967) Breakdown and Resynthesis of Phosphorylcreatine and Adenosine Triphosphate in Connection with Muscular Work in Man. Scandinavian Journal of Clinical Laboratory Investigation, 19, 56-66.

Keskinen, K.L. and Komi, P.V. (1993) Stroking Characteristics of Front Crawl Swimming during Exercise. Journal of Applied Biomechanics, 9 (3), 219-226.

32 MODELING THE EFFECTS OF TRAINING IN COMPETITIVE SWIMMING

I. MUJIKA, T. BUSSO, A. GEYSSANT, J.C. CHATARD
Laboratoire de Physiologie, GIP Exercise, Faculté de Médecine, Saint-Etienne, France

L. LACOSTE and F. BARALE
Toulouse Olympic Etudiant Club, Toulouse, France

Abstract

This study has investigated the effect of training on performance and the response to taper in elite swimmers (n = 18), with a mathematical model that links training with performance by a second order transfer function and estimates negative and positive influences of training, NI and PI. Variations in training, performance, NI and PI were studied during 3, 4 and 6 week tapers preceding three important competitions. The fit between modeled and actual performance was significant for 17 subjects (r^2 ranged from 0.45 to 0.85, $P < 0.05$). The first two tapers resulted in a significant improvement in performance: $2.94 \pm 1.51\%$ ($P < 0.01$) and $3.18 \pm 1.70\%$ ($P < 0.01$), respectively, but not the third one. NI was significantly reduced during the first two tapers ($P < 0.05$), but not during the third one. PI did not change significantly with taper. These results show that the model used is a valuable method to describe the effects of training on performance. The improvement in performance during taper was attributed to a reduction in the NI level. PI did not improve with taper, but was not compromised by the reduced training periods.

Keywords: Mathematical model, performance, systems theory, taper, training stimulus.

1 Introduction

A systems model has been proposed to study the response to training [1, 2]. According to this model, sports performance can be estimated from the difference between a negative and a positive influence representing respectively fatigue and fitness accumulated in response to training. This study aimed to investigate, using this model, the effect of training on performance and the response to taper in elite swimmers.

2 Methods

2.1 Subjects
Eighteen highly trained elite swimmers were studied (8 female, 10 male). Their mean (± SD) age, height, weight and competition background were 20.3 ± 2.8 yr, 179.0 ± 8.2 cm, 67.5 ± 11.7 kg and 11.9 ± 4.0 yr, respectively. For each swimmer, performance was measured 18 ± 3 times during the season and expressed as a percentage of the personal record achieved during the preceding season.

2.2 Quantification of the training stimulus
The training program started after detraining from the previous season and was divided into 3 main periods leading to an important competition: wk 14, 29 and 44. The training intensity was determined from blood lactate concentration and a progressive test performed in the early season. Five intensity levels were established. I: speed inferior to 2 mM; II: close to 4 mM; III: close to 6 mM; IV: high lactic swimming (10 mM); V: sprint swimming. All workouts over the season were timed for each swimmer and intensity categorized according to the five levels. Blood lactate values were measured several times throughout the season, in order to adjust the training intensity level. A stress index scale was established according to the blood lactate accumulation levels as follows: values 2, 4, 6 and 10 mM corresponded to the intensity levels I, II, III and IV, respectively. The corresponding value for intensity V was estimated as 16 mM. These values were then divided by two, in order to make them more manageable. Thus, the index scale was 1, 2, 3, 5, 8, to be multiplied by the distance swum at each intensity level. The total weekly training stimulus (W) measured in arbitrary units was computed as the sum of the number of km swum at each training intensity, multiplied by their respective weighting coefficients.

2.3 Fatigue and fitness indicators
In the systems model the athlete is considered as a system, in which the input is training and the output performance [1, 2]. The systems behavior is described by a transfer function composed of two antagonistic first order filters representing a fatiguing impulse and a fitness impulse. The model relates mathematically the resulting performance to the amount of training as the difference between fatigue and fitness. In the present study, the model performance at day n, $\hat{p}$, was calculated from the successive training loads w_i, with i varying from 1 to n-1:

$$\hat{p}_n = p* \tag{1}$$

Model performances were defined with the following model parameters: one positive and one negative multiplying factors, k_1 and k_2; one positive and one negative decay time constants, τ_1 and τ_2; and an additive term p^*, corresponding to an initial basic level of performance.   Model parameters are determined by fitting modeled performance to a real performance measured serially throughout the training program and by minimizing the residual sum of squares between them.   Fatigue and fitness indicators have been computed from the combined effects of both model functions on performance [2, 3]. These influence curves have been described in detail, in order to determine the training program that would give the best performance at a target time [4].   The sum of the negative and positive influences of training stimulus performed over the season were defined as NI and PI, respectively.

2.4 Taper
The three main competitions of the season were preceded by taper periods consisting of a progressive reduction of the amount of training and lasting 3, 4 and 6 weeks, respectively.   In order to evaluate the response of the swimmers to taper, variations in training, performance, NI and PI were studied.

2.5 Statistical analysis
Means and standard deviations or standard errors were calculated for all the variables. The statistical significance of the fit between actual performance and modeled performance was tested by an analysis of variance on the residual sum of squares. Analysis of variance (ANOVA) was used to study the variations in training, fatigue and fitness during taper.   Performance variations were evaluated with a multiple paired t - test with Bonferonni's correction.   The acceptable level of statistical significance was set at $P < 0.05$.

3 Results

3.1 Performance fit and model parameters
The fit between the actual performance at different moments of the season and the modeled performance was statistically significant for 17 of the subjects ($P < 0.05$).   The mean r^2 values of the fit were 0.65 ± 0.12 and ranged from 0.45 to 0.85.   The application of the model for one of the swimmers is presented in Figure 1.

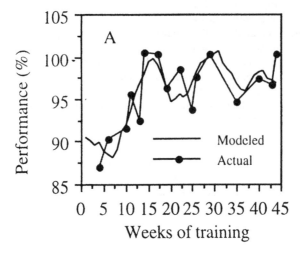

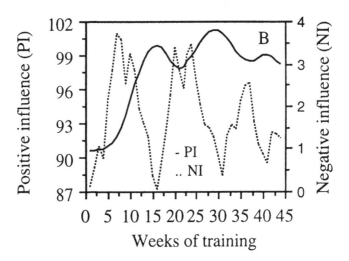

Fig. 1. Quality of the performance fit (A); NI and PI profiles (B).

3.2 Taper

The amount of training was significantly reduced during all three tapers, compared with the pre-taper training values (Fig. 2A). The first two tapers resulted in significant improvements in performance: $2.94 \pm 1.51\%$ (n = 17, $P < 0.01$) and $3.18 \pm 1.70\%$ (n = 15, $P < 0.01$), respectively (Fig. 2B). NI increased significantly from the early season to the beginning of the first taper ($P < 0.01$). Significant decrements in NI were observed during the first two tapers (Fig. 2C). PI increased significantly from the early season to

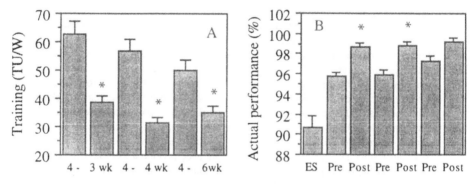

Taper 1   Taper 2   Taper 3

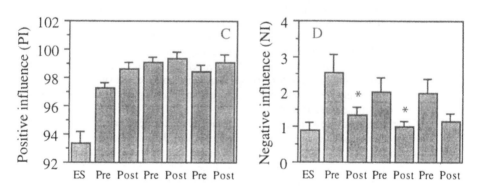

ES Taper 1 Taper 2 Taper 3

Fig. 2. Mean ($\pm$ SE) training loads (A), actual performance in % of the personal record (B), PI (C) and NI (D) at the early season (ES), between pre- and post-taper and after each taper. * denote significant differences ($P < 0.05$).

the beginning of the first taper ($P < 0.01$) and from the beginning of the first taper to the beginning of the second ($P < 0.05$), but no significant variation was observed during any of the periods of taper (Fig. 2D).

4 Discussion

The statistical significance of the performance fit confirms that the model used in the present study is a valuable method to describe the relationship between training and performance. However, an important intersubject variability was observed in the model parameter values. A great deal of this variability could probably be attributed to a lack of precision of the model, rather than to a real variability in the physical responses to training. Moreover, the precision of the model does not seem to be high enough to explain the small variations in peak performance of elite competitive swimmers. The quantification of the training load used in this study could also be too general and imprecise, since it did not take into account a great deal of other training variables used by the coaches in their programs. Furthermore, the model parameters were assumed to be constant during the entire follow-up period. Training in itself might modify the response of an athlete to a training stress [1]. Moreover, it has been shown that actual performance does not correspond to the performance predicted from model parameters fitted later in the training process, and that the follow up period should be divided into smaller periods lasting from 60 to 90 days, and the modeling process repeated in each of them [1]. This technique implies a frequency of performance measurement that is difficult to attain when studying elite swimmers. Different studies have shown the coherence of the model as a method to describe biological responses to training. Indeed, variations in iron status [5], several serum enzyme activities [1] and hormonal adaptations [3, 6] have been shown to significantly correlate with modeled fatigue and fitness indicators. Studying the individual curves reflecting fatigue and fitness could thus provide valuable information for the understanding of the individual responses to training. This would permit one to avoid overtraining and to modify the training process in order to optimize performance.

Taper intends to allow the elimination of fatigue without compromising fitness. The duration of taper should be long enough to minimize the stressing effects of training, while avoiding the fall into detraining [7]. The duration of taper would thus depend on such factors as previous training, fatigue, fitness levels and degree of the training reduction. In the present study, the swimmers tapered for 21, 28 and 42 days, and swimming performance improved by _ 3% during the first two tapers. These values were similar to those reported for competition swimmers in previous studies [8, 9, 10]. The nonsignificant improvement in performance achieved during the third taper could be explained by a low pre-taper training level and a high pre-taper performance level. This observations are justified by the fact that most of the swimmers were regularly participating in different meetings held at that time of the season, for which reasonably high levels of performance were required. The actual performance and NI followed inverse patterns during the different pre-taper and taper periods. Calvert et al. [11] suggested that fatigue function becomes more important as the athlete's fitness level reaches the upper limit of his genetically determined performance capacity. Thus, it could be suggested that during taper, improvements in performance were mainly due to significant reductions in the levels of NI, rather than to the nonsignificant variations in PI.

In conclusion, the mathematical model used in this study permitted to relate swimming training with performance and to estimate individual profiles of the negative and positive influences of training on performance. During taper, the improvement in performance was attributed to a reduction in the NI level. PI did not improve with taper, but was not compromised by the reduced training periods.

5 References

1. Banister, E.W. (1991) Modeling elite athletic performance, in *Physiological Testing of Elite Athletes*, (ed. H.J. Green, J.D. McDougal and H. Wenger), Champaign Human Kinetics Publishers, pp. 403-424.
2. Busso, T., Candau, R. and Lacour, J.R. (1994) Fatigue and fitness modelled from the effects of training on performance. *European Journal of Applied Physiology*, Vol. 69. pp. 50-54.
3. Busso, T., Hakkinen, K., Pakarinen, A., Kauhanen, H, Komi, P.V. and Lacour, J.R. (1992) Hormonal adaptations and modelled responses in elite weightlifters during 6 weeks of training. *European Journal of Applied Physiology*, Vol. 64. pp. 381-386.
4. Fitz-Clarke, J.R., Morton, R.H. and Banister E.W. (1991) Optimizing athletic perfomance by influence curves. *Journal of Applied Physiology*, Vol. 71. pp. 1151-1158.
5. Banister, E.W. and Hamilton, C.L. (1985) Variations in iron status with fatigue modelled from training in female distance runners. *European Journal of Applied Physiology*, Vol. 54. pp. 16-23.
6. Busso, T., Hakkinen, K., Pakarinen, A., Carasso, C., Lacour, J.R., Komi, P.V. and Kauhanen, H. (1990) A systems model of training responses and its relationships to hormonal responses in elite weight-lifters. *European Journal of Applied Physiology*, Vol. 61. pp. 48-54.
7. Neufer, P.D. (1989) The effect of detraining and reduced training on the physiological adaptations to aerobic exercise training. *Sports Medicine*, Vol. 8. pp. 302-321.
8. Costill, D.L., Thomas, R., Robergs, R.A., Pascoe, D., Lambert, C., Barr, S. and Fink, W.J. (1991) Adaptations to swimming training : influence of training volume. *Medicine and Science in Sports and Exercise*, Vol. 23. pp. 371-377.
9. Costill, D.L., King, D.S., Thomas, R. and Hargreaves, M. (1985) Effects of reduced training on muscular power in swimmers. *Physician and Sportsmedicine*, Vol. 13. pp. 94-101.

10. Johns, R.A., Houmard, J.A., Kobe, R.W., Hortobagyi, T., Bruno, N.J., Wells, J.M. and Shinebarger, M.H. (1992) Effects of taper on swim power, stroke distance and performance. *Medicine and Science in Sports and Exercise*, Vol. 24. pp. 1141-1146.

11. Calvert, T.W., Banister, E.W., Savage, M.V. and Bach, T. (1976) A systems model of the effects of training on physical performance. *IEEE Transactions on Systems, Man , and Cybernetics*, Vol. 6. pp. 94-102.

33 THE RELATIONSHIP BETWEEN 1500 M SWIMMING PERFORMANCE AND CRITICAL POWER USING AN ISOKINETICSWIM BENCH

I.L. SWAINE

Department of Physical education, Sport and Leisure,
De Montfort University Bedford,Bedford, UK.

Abstract

The measurement of critical power (CP) has experienced a resurgence of interest in recent years and appears to have useful application to the study of human performance. The purpose of this study was to investigate the relationship between critical power (CP), as determined using an isokinetic swim bench, and middle distance swimming performance (1500m). Twelve male competitive swimmers (age 18.4 ± 2.8 years; best time 1024 ± 86.3 s; mean, SD) gave written informed consent and were recruited to the study. The CP was determined on a computer-interfaced isokinetic swim bench (CIISB) which uses force, distance and duration transducers on individual pulley-ropes for right and left arms, to compute work done per stroke and power output. Four all-out effort tests to exhaustion, at different power output settings, were performed with 1 hr recovery. The time limit (T_{lim}) and total work done (W_{lim}) for each test were recorded and used to calculate CP, as the slope 'b' of the regression equation $W_{lim} = a + b \cdot T_{lim}$. All subjects also completed a 1500m front crawl swim time trial (TT_{1500}) on a separate occasion. The mean CP as determined on the swim bench was 120.7 ± 4.9 W (mean $\pm$ SEM) and mean TT_{1500} was 1036 ± 22.6 s. The TT_{1500} was significantly correlated with CP ($r=-0.89$; $p<0.05$) and was given by; $TT_{1500} = 1563 - 4.4 \cdot CP$ (SEE,52.1; V%,4.7). These results suggest that CP is a valuable indicator of middle-distance swimming performance in trained swimmers and that it is possible to determine CP using non-invasive techniques in the laboratory with the computer-interfaced isokinetic swim bench.

Keywords: Critical power, swim bench, 1500m time trial, swimming.

1 Introduction

Critical power (CP) was originally proposed as an index of performance-specific endurance [1]. More recently CP has been shown to correlate with the onset of blood lactate accumulation [2, 3], the individual anaerobic threshold [4] and the ventilatory threshold [5]. It has also been used to predict time to exhaustion during cycling [6] and has been shown to change in response to endurance training [7]. However, in all of these studies CP has been assessed during cycle ergometry, chiefly because it is necessary to manipulate power output. It has not been possible to measure CP in swimmers, since a swimming-specific ergometer has not been available. Nevertheless, the concept has been applied to swimming in water-based assessment of the critical velocity (V_{crit}) by Wakoyoshi et al. [8] who found this index to correlate well with 400m swimming performance.

The CP is determined by elucidation of the slope 'b' in the linear plot of total work done (W_{lim}) against time limit (T_{lim}) for a series of maximal exercise bouts at different power output settings. Recent advances in development of the computer-interfaced isokinetic swim bench (CIISB) have meant that power output during simulated swimming can be determined and manipulated. Tranducers on the pulley ropes allow measurement of pull force, distance and duration which can be computed to give power output and a simple visual display scale allows the subject to maintain a predetermined level. The purpose of this study was to explore the relationship between CP, as determined on the CIISB, and endurance (1500 m) swimming performance.

2 Methods

Twelve male competitive swimmers gave informed consent and were recruited to the study. Their average age was 18.4± 2.8 years; body mass 74.7±2.9 kg and stature 1.79± 0.04 m (mean ± SD). All were involved in swimming training for 1.5 hours at least 7 times per week for 6 months prior to the study. All subjects attended the laboratory for assessment after having refrained from exercise training for 24 hours. The CP was determined by regression of the T_{lim} vs. W_{lim} plot for four separate bouts of exercise on the CIISB (H and M. Engineering, Gwent, Wales). This method was adapted from Monod and Scherrer [1].

The use of the CIISB has previously been described in detail [9]. Subjects adopted a prone posture and simulated the front crawl arm action. Force was exerted alternately on hand pulleys which pulled-out at a fixed maximal velocity [10]. The pulley ropes were passed through transducers which measured pull -force, -distance and -duration, from which mean power output was computed. Subjects were instructed to maintain a given power output (W) by use of a pointer-scale on a visual display unit. The software used with this ergometer was written specifically for exercise testing (H. Smith, University of Sunderland, 1992). Four bouts of exercise were used at 100, 125, 150 and

175 W. Subjects were instructed to exercise until exhaustion and the W_{lim} and T_{lim} were recorded. A recovery period of one hour was allowed between each exercise bout.

3 Results

The mean value for CP was 120.7, 9.4 W (mean, SD). All subjects displayed a linear relationship when the four exercise test values of W_{lim} and T_{lim} were plotted (at least r=0.998; p=0.001). The mean time for TT_{1500} was 1036, 74.6 s. The TT_{1500} was significantly correlated (r=0.899; p=0.01) with best time. The relationship between CP and TT_{1500} was significant (r=-0.89; p<0.05) and the regression equation was given by TT_{1500} = 1563 - 4.4·CP (SEE, 52.1; V%,4.7).

4 Discussion

The significant relationship between CP and swimming performance contrasts with other exercise test indices determined on this ergometer [9]. Cardiopulmonary indices such as VO_2max, ventilatory threshold (VT) and peak exercise intensity from a continuous incremental ramp test showed insignificant correlation with 400m swimming performance. Other workers have found a significant relationship between VO_2max and swimming performance [11], using an arm ergometer, for a heterogeneous group. However, the study of Swaine [9] involved a homogeneous group of swimmers which had small differences in performance.

The presence of a significant relationship between swim bench exercise test indices and swimming performance for 1500m, where none apparently exists for 400m, might be explained by the relative contribution of the arms to overall propulsion in the two events. There is a greater contribution to propulsion from the legs in 400m as compared to 1500m swimming [12] which might reduce the correlation between arms-only indices from the swim bench and swimming performance.

The results of this study show that it is possible to accurately determine critical power in swimmers using the CIISB. All relationships of W_{lim} and T_{lim} showed high correlation. Of additional interest is that the CP assessment procedure also allows the elucidation of an index of anaerobic capacity. This is given by the intercept 'y' of the regression line W_{lim} vs T_{lim}. Such an index has been shown to provide an indication of the capacity for repeated maximal intensity exercise [13]. A similar index has been validated [14] and found to be of value in assessment of differences in anaerobic power of age-group swimmers [15]. Clearly, this simple non-invasive procedure using the CIISB could provide comprehensive assessment of swimming-specific metabolism which appears to correlate well with swimming performance. Furthermore, since these power indices have been shown to detect changes associated with training [7, 16], they may be of value in studies of metabolism in swimmers during training.

5 References

1. Monod, H. and Scherrer, J. (1965) The work capacity of a synergic muscular group. *Ergonomics*, 8:329-337.
2. Jenkins, G.J. and Quigley, B.M. (1990) Blood lactate in trained cyclists during cycle ergometry at critical power. *European Journal of Applied Physiology*, 61:278-283.
3. Housh, T.J., Devries, H.A., Housh, D.J., Tichy, M.W., Smyth, K.D., and Tichy, A.M. (1991) The relationship between critical power and the onset of blood lactate accumulation. *Journal of Sports Medicine and Physical Fitness*, 31: 31-36.
4. McLellan, T.M. and Cheung K.S.Y. (1992) A comparitive evaluation of the individual anaeriobic threshold and the critical power. *Medicine and Science in Sports and Exercise*, 24: 329-337.
5. Moritani, T., Nagata, A., DeVries, H.A. and Muro, M. (1981) Critical power as a measure of physical work capacity and anaerobic threshold. *Ergonomics*, 24: 339-350.
6. Housh, D.J., Housh, T.J. and Bauge, S.M. (1989) The accuracy of the critical power test for predicting time to exhaustion during cycle ergometry. *Ergonomics*, 32:997-1004.
7. Jenkins, G.J. and Quigley B.M. (1992) Endurance training enhances critical power. *Medicine and Science in Sports and Exercise*, 24(11): 1283-1289.
8. Wakayoshi K., Ikuta, K., Yoshida, T., Udo, M., Moritani, T., Mutch, Y. and Miyashita, M. (1992) Determination and validity of critical velocity as an index of swimming performance in the competitive swimmer. *European Journal of Applied Physiology and Occupational Physiology*, 64(2): 153-157.
9. Swaine I.L. (1994) The relationship between physiological variables from a swim bench ramp test and middle-distance swimming performance. *Journal of Swimming Research*. In press.
10. Sharp, R. L., Troup, J. P. and Costill, D.L. (1982) Relationship between power and sprint freestyle swimming. *Medicine and Science in Sports and Exercise*, 14(1): 53-56.
11. Obert, P., Failgairette, G., Bedu, M. and Coudert, J. (1992) Bioenergetic characteristics of swimmers determined during an arm-ergometer test and during swimming. *International Journal of Sports Medicine*, 13(4): 298-303.
12. Hollander, A.P., de Groot, G., van Ingen Schenau, G.J., Kahman, R. and Toussaint H. (1988) Contribution of the legs to propulsion in front crawl swimming. In *Swimming Science V*. Ungerechts, B.E., Wilke, K. and Reischle, K. (eds). Human Kinetics Books. Champaign, Ill. pp 39-45.
13. Jenkins, G.J. and Quigley, B.M. (1990) The y-intercept of the critical power function as a measure of anaerobic work capacity. *Ergonomics*, 34: 13-22.

14. Takahashi, S., Bone, M., Cappaert, J.M., Barzdukas, A., D'Acquisto, L., Hollander, A.P. and Troup, J. P. (1992a) Validation of a dryland swimming specific measurement of anaerobic power. In *Biomechanics and Medicine in Swimming VI*. Maclaren, D., Reilly T. and Lees A. (eds). E. and F. N. Spon. London. pp 301-305.

15. Takahashi, S., Bone, M., Spry, S., Trappe, S. and Troup, J. P. (1992b) Differences in the anaerobic power of age group swimmers. In *Biomechanics and Medicine in Swimming VI*. Maclaren, D., Reilly, T. and Lees A. (eds). E. and F. N. Spon. London. pp 289-294.

16. Jenkins, G.J. and Quigley, B.M. (1993) The influence of high-intensity exercise training on the W-T relationship. *Medicine and Science in Sports and Exercise*, 25(2): 275-282.

Acknowledgements

This work was supported by the *Institute of Swimming Teachers and Coaches, The Sports Council* and *The City of Leeds Swimming Scheme*.

34 GROWTH AND DEVELOPMENTAL CHANGES IN SELECTED CHARACTERISTICS OF ELITE AGE GROUP SWIMMERS

S.A. KAVOURAS and J.P. TROUP

United States Swimming, International Center for Aquatic Research, U.S. Olympic Training Center, Colorado Springs, USA.

Abstract

This investigation had two objectives: 1) to determine when significant maturation occurs in young elite swimmers and 2) to determine developmental differences in morphological and physiological characteristics. Three year longitudinal (L) and cross-sectional data (CS) were collected. All subjects were top 10 in the United States for their age group (ages: 13 - 17, and 14 - 18, for females and males, respectively). For the L and CS design 64 (males=32; females=32), and 960 (males=480 ; females=480) swimmers were tested. All the testing was done during the same time of the year, and during the same phase of training, in organized training camp. Tests conducted were: a) anthropometrics, b) strength, c) aerobic and anaerobic capacity, and d) performance time trials. Peak growth velocity (PGV) for height and body segments were between 14-16 (males) and 13-14 (females). PGV's for muscle area and strength were between 14-15 (females) and 15-16 (males). Maximal oxygen consumption PGV was between 14-15 for the females with no significant increase after the age of 16 ($p > 0.05$). The same parameter for males showed PGV between 15-16 and did not change after the age of 17 ($p > 0.05$). Anaerobic capacity growth rate peaked after the age of 15 for both males and females and did not plateau until the age of 17 and 18 for males and females, respectively. This information can be used to design developmentally specific training programs.

1. Introduction

Physiological and morphological changes in children during puberty are well documented (10). Body size, strength, as well as aerobic and anaerobic capacities increase due to maturation (3,6,7,13). Those parameters will also improve with training, but the degree of improvement in strength and anaerobic capacity is smaller in children than in adults (1,9,15). However there is very little information of the interaction effect of maturation and training in elite young swimmers (2).

The purpose of this study was: 1) to determine when significant maturation occurs in young elite swimmers, and 2) to determine at what age different morphological and physiological characteristics develop the most. This information could be useful for the design of appropriate training programs for age group swimmers.

2. Methods

2.1 Subjects

The study included two designs, for analysis of developmental changes: one longitudinal (L), and one cross-sectional (CS). For the L design, the same 64 subjects (32 males and 32 females) were tested once a year for three consecutive years. For the CS design, a total of 960 subjects (480 males and 480 females) participated throughout the course of three years. The age for the males and females was 14 to 18 and 13 to 17, respectively. The same number of subjects were used for each age, and gender group (N=96 each). Subjects were informed of the experimental procedure, and the risk associated with the experiment. In addition, written consents were obtained for each one, according to IRB procedures of U.S. Swimming. The subjects were year round competitive swimmers, ranked top ten in the United States for their age group (none swimmers were national or junior national team). All testing was done during the same time of the year in an organized training camp, at the International Center for Aquatic Research, in Colorado Springs, CO (altitude: 1870 m), between 1990 and 1993.

2.2 Muscle Area:

The term muscle area (MA) refers to the upper arm cross sectional muscle and bone area. This parameter was derived upon girth and skinfold measurement. For the purpose of this study, MA was calculated (cm^2) using the following formula (8):

$$MA=[ArmG-0.1\pi(Tri+Bi)]^2/4\pi \qquad (Kavouras, 92)$$

MA: muscle and bone cross sectional area expressed in cm^2.
ArmG: relaxed upper arm girth, measured in cm, when subject is in standing
*   position with arm in abduction at 90° with elbow at 90°.*
π: geometrical standard 3.14.
Tri: triceps skinfold, measured in mm.
Bi: biceps skinfold, measured in mm.

2.3 Muscle Power

In order to measure upper body muscle power, a computerized Pacer 2A Biokinetics swimming ergometer (Isokinetics Inc) was used. Each subject completed a series of three double arm pulls (butterfly pull) through full range of motion, while prone, at four different settings (0, 3, 6, and 9). The peak power from these trials was used as muscle power.

2.4 Maximal Oxygen Consumption (VO_2max)

Maximal oxygen consumption during freestyle swimming was measured, using a swimming treadmill, as an indicator of aerobic capacity. This test consisted of a two minute swim, at a pace approximately 1.15 m/sec (corresponding to 70-80 % of the subjects best 200m freestyle time). After this time, the water speed was increased by 0.05 m/sec for every 30 seconds, until volitional exhaustion occurred. During the test, expired gases were continuously sampled from a mixing chamber and analyzed on line at 10 sec intervals via applied electrochemistry (Ametek), which was interfaced to an IBM computer. To determine the maximal oxygen consumption, the three highest consecutive readings were averaged.

2.5 Maximal Oxygen Deficit

This test was completed on the day after the VO_2max test. During that test, subjects swam at the velocity corresponding to 100% of the maximal oxygen uptake until volitional exhaustion. During that time, the oxygen uptake was recorded continuously. The accumulated oxygen uptake was calculated on 30 sec intervals. The absolute difference between the estimated oxygen demand (5), and the accumulated oxygen uptake was defined as the accumulated oxygen deficit (11). It has been found that O_2 deficit measured this way is an accurate indicator of anaerobic power (11).

2.6 Swimming Performance

Swimming times were provided as current best-time, by the United States Swimming. Those times were converted into a score value based on the FINA swimming performance scoring system. Using this method, swimming performance of different stoke or distances could be compared.

2.7 Rate of Change

Data in the graphs are expressed as the mean change of each variables from year to year. Those data are derived from subtraction of the absolute value of a variable for each year from the previous one. Since the rate of change between the CS and L study designs did not differ significantly ($p>0.05$), the graphs represent the values of the CS design.

2.8 Statistics

For the CS design, variables were analyzed using one way analysis of variance (ANOVA) for repeated measures. For the L design, variables were analyzed using one way analysis of variance (ANOVA) for repeated measures. Comparisons in the rates of change between the CS and the L design were done by analysis of variance (ANOVA). Significant differences between the means were determined by using Tukey's post-hoc analysis, accepted at the $p< 0.05$ level. Curve fitting was derived from a third degree polynomial.

3. Results

Height as well as body segments were measured in this investigation. We found that the rate of increase for males peaked between the ages of 14 and 16, with no significant increase after the age of 17. In females, peak height velocity was found between the ages of 13 and 14. In the height graph (Figure 1) appears that peak height velocity for females occurred, probably, before the age of 13.

The fat free, muscle and bone area of the upper arm, was found to increase significantly for every year between the ages of 14 to 18 and 14 to 16 for males and females, respectively. The muscle area peak growth velocity was evident between the age of 15 to 16 for males and 14 to 15 for females.

Males peak growth velocity in muscle power, appeared at the age range 15 to 16, with statistically significant increased up to 18 years. Similarly, females showed peak growth velocity for muscle power in the ages of 13 to 15, with no plateau until the age of 17.

Swimming aerobic capacity, measured as absolute maximal oxygen consumption in a swimming treadmill, showed the following results: Males and females peak growth velocity, occurred between the ages of 15 to 16 and 14 to 15, respectively. Interestingly, no further significant increase occurred after the age of 17 for males and after the age of 16 for females.

Swimming anaerobic capacity, measured as maximal accumulated oxygen deficit, demonstrated no significant increase before the age of 15 and 14 for males and females, respectively. After the aforementioned, ages maximal accumulated oxygen deficit increased continuously and no plateau appeared for males (until the age of 18) or females (until the age of 17). Peak growth velocity for anaerobic capacity was evident for males, at the age of 16 to 17, and for females, at the age of 15 to 16.

TABLE 2. *Age that males and females achieved their peak growth velocity and peak growth (plateau). NA means that plateau at that given characteristic was not evident.*

	Peak Growth Velocity		Peak Growth (plateau)	
	Males	**Females**	**Males**	**Females**
Height	14-16	13-14	17>	15>
Muscle Area	15-16	14-15	NA	16>
Muscle Power	15-16	13-15	NA	NA
VO$_2$max	15-16	14-15	17>	16>
O$_2$ Deficit	16-17	15-16	NA	NA

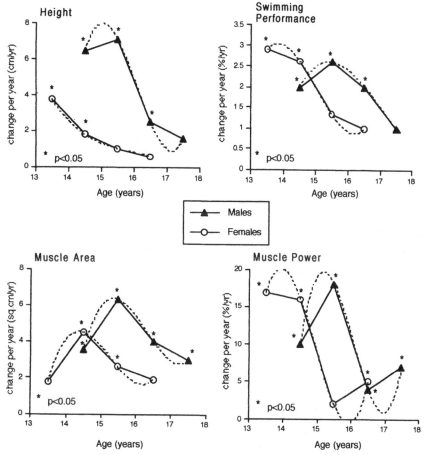

FIGURE 1. *Rate of improvement of height, swimming performance, muscle area, and muscle power from year to year for males (▲) and females (O). The * indicates statistically significant change from the previous year at p level 0.05.*

4. Discussion

The purposes of this investigation were primarily, to identify when significant maturation occurs, and, secondary, to distinguish the age at which different morphological and physiological parameters appear to develop at a faster rate. This information is useful when designing training programs specifically for age group development.

Tanner et al (13) reported peak height velocity for non-athletes males and females at the age of 14 and 12, respectively. Our data showed peak height velocity (males: 15; females: 13-14) to be reached approximately one year after. These data, as from the Tanner's study, showed height growth plateau was reached at the same age (females: 15; males: 17). In 1981, Johnson et al (6) measured the arm circumference from the ages of 2 up to 18. They found that males and females exhibit their peak growth velocity in the ages

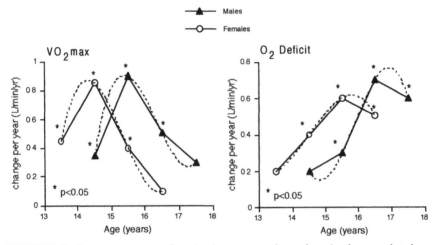

FIGURE 2. *Improvement rate of maximal oxygen uptake, and maximal accumulated oxygen deficit from year to year in males (▲) and females (O). The * indicates statistically significant change from the previous year at p level 0.05. Data for the VO₂max and O₂ deficit were based on the L subjects tested once.*

of 12 to 14 and 11 to 12, respectively. They also found that the plateau in growth appeared at the age of 15 for females, whereas males did not show a plateau up to the age of 18. Our data showed peak growth velocity for muscle area between the age of 15 to 16 (males) and 14 to 15 (females). Similarly to Johnson plateau for muscle area was not evident until the age of 18, for males. Jones (7) measured the pulling strength of shoulder in males and females between the ages of 11 to 18 and he found rapid increase in strength for males between the ages of 14 to 18, but the females demonstrate a plateau after the age of 17. In our study, no plateau was found for males or females. In 1980, Cameron et al (3), presented aerobic capacity data from boys, expressed as velocity curve of VO₂max, and he found the peak growth velocity between the ages 13 and 15 and a plateau in aerobic capacity development after the age of 16. Recently, Takahashi et al (12), measured anaerobic capacity through maximal accumulated oxygen deficit in age group swimmers. They reported an increase in anaerobic capacity after the age of 13 and subsequent increase even up to the age of 18.

Our findings, based on highly trained young elite swimmers are in agreement with the literature. In some characteristics such as muscle area our data showed a peak growth velocity at an older age, phenomenon that could be related to the training effect.

5. Conclusion

In conclusion, our data suggested: (1) elite age group swimmers appeared to be well-developed physically by the age of 16 and they are probably ready for strenuous training, (2) since muscle power and anaerobic capacity did not reach any plateau by the age of 17 or 18, there may be potential for further improvement in muscle power and anaerobic capacity. Those improvements could affect the capacity of improvement in performance (14).

6. References

1. **Atomi, Y., T. Fukunaga, Y. Yamamoto, and H. Hatta**. Lactate threshold and VO₂max of trained and untrained boys relatively to body mass and composition. In Tutenfranz, J., R. Mocellin, and F. Klimt (Eds.), *Children and Exercise XII* (pp. 53-65). Champaign, IL: Human Kinetics Publishers, 1986.
2. **Boulgakova, N.** *Selection et preparation des jeunes nageurs.* Paris: Vigot, 1990.
3. **Cameron, N., R.L. Mirwarld, and D.A. Bailey**. Standards for the assessment of normal absolute maximal aerobic power. In Ostyn, M., G. Beunen, and J. Simon (Eds.), *Kinanthropometry II* (pp. 355-358). Baltimore: University Park Press, 1980.
4. **Carter, J. E. L., and T. R. Ackland** (Eds.). *Kinanthropometry in Swimming.* Champaign, IL: Human Kinetics Publishers, 1994.
5. **Hermansen, L.** Anaerobic energy release. *Med. Scil. Sports Exerc.,* 1: 32-38, 1969.
6. **Johnson, W. R., R. Fulwood, S. Abraham, and J. D. Bryner**. Basic data on anthropometric measurements and angular measurements of the hip and knee joints for selected age groups 1-74 years of age, United States, 1971-1975. *Vital and Health Statistics,* Series 11, 1981.
7. **Jones, H. E.** *Motor performance and growth: A developmental study of static dynamometric strength.* Berkeley: University of California Press, 1949.
8. **Kavouras, S.** (Ed.). *Developmental Stages of Competitive Swimmers.* Colorado Springs, CO: U.S. Swimming, 1992.
9. **Kich, G., and L. Fransson**. Essential cardiovascular and respiratory determinants of physical performance at age 12 to 17 years during intensive physical training. In Tutenfranz, J., R. Mocellin, and F. Klimt (Eds.), *Children and Exercise XII* (pp. 275-292). Champaign, IL: Human Kinetics Publishers, 1986.
10. **Malina, R. M., and C. Bouchard.** *Growth maturation and physical activity.* Champaign, IL: Human Kinetics Publishers, 1991.
11. **Medbø, J. I., A. C. Mohn, I. Tabata, R. Bahr, O. Vaage, and O. M. Sejersted**. Anaerobic capacity determined by maximal accumulated O₂ deficit. *J. Appl. Physiol.,* 64: 50-60, 1988.

12. **Takahashi, S., M. Bone, S. Spry, S. Trappe, and J. P. Troup**. Differences in the anaerobic power of age group swimmers. In MacLaren, D., T. Reilly, and A. Lees (Eds.), *Biomechanics and Medicine in Swimming. Swimming Science VI* (pp. 289-294). London: E & FN Spon, 1992.

13. **Tanner, J. M., R. H. Whitehouse, and M. Takaishi**. Standards from birth to maturity for height, weight, height velocity, and weight velocity: British children, 1965-I. *Archives of Disease in Childhood*, 41: 454-471, 1966.

14. **Troup, J. P., D. Strass, and T. A. Trappe**. Physiology and Nutrition of Swimming. In Lamb, D. R., H. G. Knuttgen, and R. Murray (Eds.), *Physiology and Nutrition for Competitive Sport* (pp. 99-129). Carmel, IN: Cooper, 1994.

15. **Vos, J. A., W. Geurts, T. Brandon, and A. R. Binkhorst**. A logitudinal study of muscular strength and cardiorespiratory fitness in girls (13 to 18 years). In Tutenfranz, J., R. Mocellin, and F. Klimt (Eds.), *Children and Exercise XII* (pp. 233-243). Champaign, IL: Human Kinetics Publishers, 1986.

35 ENERGY EXPENDITURE OF ELITE FEMALE SWIMMERS DURING HEAVY TRAINING AND TAPER

J.L. VAN HEEST

United States Swimming, International Center for Aquatic Research, U.S. Olympic Training Center, Colorado Springs, USA.

Abstract

Assessment of energy expenditure at various times during swim training in free-living athletes has been extremely difficult. Utilization of the doubly labeled water technique enables non-invasive assessment of energy output. The present study was designed to assess whether or not energy expenditure varied at two distinct training times (heavy training and taper) within a collegiate season. Four female Division II collegiate swimmers were used as subjects in the present study. Each subject received a dose of 0.3g $H_2^{18}O$/kg and 0.75g ^2H_2O/kg estimated body water on day zero of both phases of the study. Saliva samples were collected a twenty-four hour intervals for the subsequent five days. All samples were frozen and stored until analysis. Diet records and workout logs were collected daily throughout the study. Caloric intake was determined from the food records. Energy expenditure was calculated from the carbon dioxide and respiratory quotient with subsequent determination of fat mass and fat free mass for each subject. Due to the small sample size, trend analysis between phases was utilized.
Keywords: Swimming, energy balance, doubly labeled water.

1 Introduction

Understanding the energy expended during training is critical to developing an optimal caloric intake to maintain body composition and maximize training in female athletes. To date, research is limited which provides information regarding energy expenditure during swim training. This is due to the technical difficulties in measuring energy expenditure in this population.   Researchers have used the backward extrapolation of oxygen consumption during recovery to estimate energy expenditure during the event (1,2). Recently, scientists have used doubly labled water to assess energy expenditure in female swimmers (3). The doubly labeled water technique appears to be useful in the evaluation of athlete groups such as swimmers.   Therefore, the present study was designed to evaluate the energy expediture at two specific times during a competitive swim season. The evaluation times are immediately prior to taper (heavy training) and during the final week of taper. The purpose of this work was to compare the energy cost associated with these types of training in female collegiate swimmers. Moreover, the results should provide information which would allow the development of optimal training regimes during these periods.

2 Methods

2.1 Subjects and Diets
Four female collegiate (Division II) swimmers served as subjects.   The women all qualified for post season National level competition, therefore these were highly competitive athletes. They reported no history of cardiovascular or metabolic disease. All procedures complied with Human Subjects regulations at the International Center for Aquatic Research.   Moreover, all subjects signed an inform consent form prior to participation in the study. The women were assessed on two seperate occasions, once during heavy training and once at the end of taper. Training regimes for the subjects were controlled by the head coach and were monitored throughout each assessment phase. During each phase, the subjects maintained dietary records. Subjects received oral instructions for determining portion size and reporting techniques on the diet logs. The diet reports were collected daily by the primary investigator. The food quotent, diet composition and caloric intake were determined for each swimmer.

2.2 Energy Expenditure and Body Composition
Baseline saliva samples were collected prior to the administration of oral doses of 0.3g $H_2{}^{18}O$/kg and 0.75g $^{2}H_2O$/kg estimated body water. Saliva samples were collected 8, 24,48,72,96, and 120 hours following dose administration for measurement of enrichment. Subjects were instructed regarding the collection and handling of the saliva samples. The samples were stored in sealed cryotubes at -50 degrees C. until analysis. All samples were analyzed for the stable isotope on a mass spectrometer. Natural log decay slopes were determined from the enrichment data.   Caloric expenditure was calculated from the carbon dioxide production rate and the food quotents for all subjects. Fat mass (FM) and fat free mass (FFM) were determined by skinfold measures and ^{18}O dilution space during each phase of the study. Body composition was calculated from the skinfold measures. Due to the small sample size, the investigators determined that no

statistical calculations would be used for the data. Descriptive statistics will be reported. In addition, trend analysis will be used to describe the results.

3 Results

The subjects were 20.75±0.5 years in age. Height ranged between 172.1 and 189.2 cm. The average body weight was 67.3±4.65 kg during heavy training and 66.12±2.74 kg during taper. Diet composition for each evaluation period (heavy training;HT and taper;TA) are displayed in Table 1. Composition of the diet remained relatively constant between the two phases.

Table 1. Composition of Diet

Subject/Phase		Food Quotent	% Fat	% Protein	% Carbohydrate
One	HT	0.92	16	16	68
	TA	0.92	17	16	67
Two	HT	0.91	22	14	64
	TA	0.91	17	11	71
Three	HT	0.90	26	12.5	60.5
	TA	0.89	26	12	62
Four	HT	0.90	26	16	59
	TA	0.90	27	17	59

Workout distance was greater during the heavy training phase compared to the taper phase (Figure 1). Average training distance during heavy training was approximately two times greater than during taper. Evaluation of the compartmental changes in body composition determined using the doubly labeled water technique indicated that three of the women increased FFM during the taper period compared to heavy training (Figure 2). In addition, all subjects lost FM during taper compared to heavy training. Figure 3 illustrates reported energy intake and energy expenditure (TEE) calculated from the results of the doubly labeled water. The subjects were not in energy balance during either phase of the study. Subjects One and Two had similar trends in both intake and TEE data. These women consumed more calories during heavy training than during taper and expended more calories during taper compared to heavy training. Subjects Three and Four had TEE that was greater during heavy training versus taper.

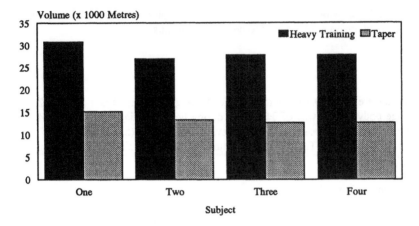

Figure 1. Workout Distances

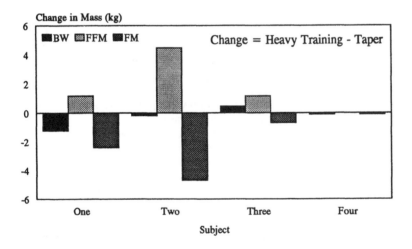

Figure 2. Changes in Body Composition

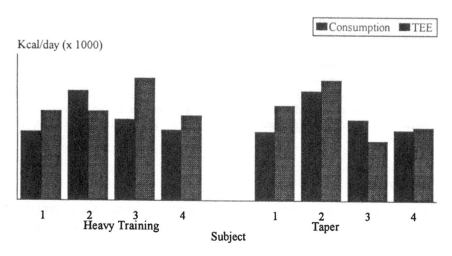

Figure 3. Energy Intake and Energy Expenditure

4 Discussion

In light of limited sample size, the results of this study must be viewed with caution. However, review of trends in the current data supports the following comments.

Three of the four women were in negative energy balance during both phases of the study. The other subject was in negative energy balance during taper and positive balance during heavy training. These results lead to the speculation that female athlete have high energy efficiency thereby allowing for an imbalance between consumption and output. The concept of "energy efficiency" has been reported previously in other trained female populations (3,4,5,6). However, the concept of "energy efficiency" is controversial. Horton et al. (7) evaluated trained cyclists compared to lean control women using whole-room indirect calorimetry. Under these conditions of tight control, the authors report that the speculated "energy efficiency" was not evident (7). The differences in energy intake versus energy output seen in the present study may be a function of inaccurate dietary recall by the subjects investigated. However, altered metabolic function and/or differences in substrate oxidation in swimmers may be present that are not seen in land based athletes. Competitive swimmers certainly would not be considered as obese, however, they tend to preserve body fat despite the high level of training they undergo daily. Swimmers might possess alterations in the utilization of fuels both during exercise and during recovery might be affected by the type of training (long duration of repeated high intensity work bouts), potential alterations in thermoregulatory mechanisms due to training in water, or the multiple cycling of training throughout the year. A combination of these mechanisms could also be plausible. It could be possible that female swimmers preferentially use carbohydrates for fuel thereby sparing the dietary fat intake that is ultimately stored as body fat.

The data indicate that competitive female swimmers have a higher energy intake during heavy training than during taper. However, these subjects were able to maintain overall body weight during the taper phase. It might be due to the reduction in caloric intake during the taper period by these women although the absolute differences in calories does not support this concept.

It appears that the doubly labeled water technique appears to be a useful tool to indicate the energy expenditure in swimmers. This method should be used in future research to investigate additional questions in energy balance during competitive swimming.

5 References

1. COSTILL, D.L., J. KOVALESKI, D. PORTER, J. KIRWAN, R. FIELDING, AND D. KING. (1985) Energy expenditure during front crawl swimming: predicting success in middle-distance events. *International Journal Sports Medicine* 6:266-270.

2. COSTILL, D.L., R. THOMAS, R.A. ROBERGS, D. PASCOE, C. LAMBERT, S. BARR, AND W.J. FINK. (1991) Adaptations to swimming training: influence of training volume. *Medicine and Science in Sports Exercise* 23:371-377.

3. JONES, P.J., and C.A. LEITCH. (1993) Validation of doubly labeled water for measurement of caloric expenditure in collegiate swimmers. *Journal of Applied Physiology* 74(6):2909-2914.

4. PATE, R.R., R.G. SARGENT, C. BALDWIN, and M.L. BURGESS. Dietary intake of women runners. (1990) *International Journal of Sports Medicine* 11:461-466.

5. SCHULTZ, L.O., S. ALGER, I. HARPER, J.H. WILMORE, and E. RAVUSSIM, (1992) Energy expenditure of elite female runners measured by respiratory chamber and doubly labeled water. *Journal of Applied Physiology* 72(1):23-28.

6. SNEAD, B.B., C.C. STUBBS, J.Y. WELTMAN, W.S. EVANS, J.D. VELDHUIS, A.D. ROGOL, C.D. TEATES, and A. WELTMAN. (1992) Dietary patterns, eating behaviors, and bone mineral density in women runners. *American Journal of Clinical Nutrition* 56:705-711.

7. HORTON, T.J., H.J. DROUGAS, T.A. SHARP, L.R. MARTINEZ, G.W. REED, and J.O. HILL. (1994) Energy balance in endurance-trained female cyclists and untrained controls. *Journal of Applied Physiology* 76(5):1937-1945.

36 ELECTRICAL STIMULATION OF THE LATISSIMUS DORSI IN SPRINT SWIMMERS
Electrical stimulation in swimming

F. PICHON, A. MARTIN, G. COMETTI
Groupe Analyse du Mouvement, UFR STAPS, Université de Bourgogne, Dijon, France

J.C. CHATARD
Laboratoire de Physiologie, GIP Exercice, Faculté de Médecine, St-Etienne, France

Abstract
The influence of a 3-wk period of electrostimulation training on the strength of the latissimus dorsi and the performances of 14 competitive swimmers divided into 7 electrostimulated (EG) and 7 control swimmers (CG) was studied. The peak torque registered during the flexion-extension of the arm was determined with an isokinetic dynamometer at velocities from $-60 °s^{-1}$ to $360 °s^{-1}$. Performances were measured over a 25-m pull buoy and a 50-m freestyle swim. For EG, a significant increase of the peak torque was measured in isometric, eccentric and concentric conditions ($P < 0.05$). The swimming times declined significantly ($P < 0.01$) by 0.19 ± 0.14 s, for the 25-m pull-buoy, and by 0.38 ± 0.24 s, for the 50-m freestyle. For CG, no significant difference was found for any of the tests. For the whole group, the variations of the peak torques, measured in eccentric condition ($-60 °s^{-1}$) were related to the variations of the performances ($r = 0.77$; $P < 0.01$). These results showed that an electrostimulation program of the latissimus dorsi increased the strength and performances of a group of competitive swimmers.
Keywords: Electrical stimulation, isokinetic dynamometer, latissimus dorsi, strength training, stroke length, stroke rate, performance.

1 Introduction

Electrostimulation is a technique of muscle strengthening based on the electrical stimulation of intramuscular branches of motor nerves which induces muscular contraction. This technique has been demonstrated to improve the isometric strength of the quadriceps femoris muscle for patients and recently, it was used as a strengthening means in the training program of athletes [1]. Gains ranging from 0% [2] to 44% [1] has been reported. However, no study has been carried out in swimming although muscle strength has been shown to be an important factor of success on short distances [3, 4, 5]. Thus, the purpose of the present study was to assess the influence of a 3-wk period of electrostimulation on the strength of the latissimus dorsi of a group of competitive swimmers and to determine whether the improvement in muscular strength from dryland training could result in faster swimming performances. The latissimus dorsi was chosen because it has been demonstrated to be extensively involved in swimming [6] and because it can be easily electrostimulated as it is a superficial muscle.

2 Methods

2.1 Subjects
A group of 14 competitive swimmers was studied. All the swimmers were sprinters, 50 or 100-m freestyle specialists. They were divided into 2 groups : 7 electrostimulated (EG) and 7 control swimmers (CG). Their main characteristics are summarized in Table 1.

Table 1. Mean (SD) characteristics of the swimmers.

	Age (yr)	Height (cm)	Weight (kg)	50-m best time (s)	Training duration (h/w)
Electrostimulated	23 (2.1)	179 (5.3)	72,8 (6.5)	25.30 (0.68)	8.5 (1.6)
Control	23 (2.3)	178 (6.0)	75 (7.8)	26.95 (2.23)	8.5 (1.6)

No significant difference was found between the mean values of the two groups.

2.2 Electrostimulation training
It was carried out over a 3-wk period, 12 min per session, 3 sessions per wk. Electrostimulation was performed with a Stiwell® stimulator and a pulse currents of 80 Hz frequency lasting 300 µs. The contraction time was 6 s and the rest time 20 s. The number of contractions per session was 27. All the swimmers used a Myostatic® dynamometer to control by themselves the intensity of the muscle contraction planned to correspond to 60% of the maximal voluntary contraction.

2.3 Measurement of muscle strength
The peak torque of the flexion-extension of the dominant arm was measured before and after training with an isokinetic dynamometer, Biodex®, at -60 °s^{-1}, 0 °s^{-1}, 60 °s^{-1}, 120 °s^{-1}, 180 °s^{-1}, 240 °s^{-1}, 300 °s^{-1} , and 360 °s^{-1} which were performed in a randomized order. Each velocity was repeated twice with a 4-min rest. Only the best performance was retained. In isometric action, the effort lasted 5 s and a 1-min period of rest separated the repetitions. The shoulder angle was 140 ° (0 ° corresponding at the complete extension of the arm).

2.4 Swimming performances
They were measured in a 25-m pool. The first test was a 25-m swim with the arms only. A pull-buoy was held between the thighs and a belt fastened to the ankles avoided the use of the legs during swimming (25PB). The second swim was a 50-m whole stroke freestyle (50FS). The two swims were performed starting in the water, without diving. The 50FS swim was videoed and the stroke rate was measured with a frequency meter. The stroke length was calculated by dividing the mean velocity of the whole swim by the stroke rate.

2.5 Statistical analysis
Means and standard deviations were calculated for all the variables. Analyses of variance (ANOVA) were used to compare the main characteristics, performances, muscular strength, stroke length and stroke rate of the two groups (EG and CG) and Student's "t" test was used to compare the effects of the electrostimulation program on

strength, performances, and biomechanical parameters. For the whole group, correlation coefficients were calculated between the variations of the peak torques and the variations of performances. In all the statistical analyses, the 0.05 level of significance was adopted.

3 Results

3.1 Effect of electrostimulation on muscle strength
For EG (Fig.1), peak torques increased significantly in isometric (+21%; P < 0.01), eccentric (+24,1% at -60 $°s^{-1}$; P < 0.01) and concentric conditions (+10.3% at 180 $°s^{-1}$; P < 0.02; +14.4% at 300 $°s^{-1}$; P < 0.03; and +14.7% at 360 $°s^{-1}$; P < 0.04). For CG, no significant difference was observed.

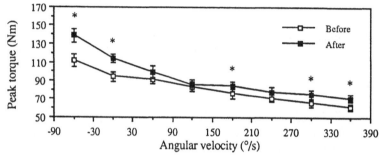

Fig. 1. Relationship between the peak torque and the angular velocity before and after training for the electrostimulated group, * denotes significance, (P < 0.05).

3.2 Effect of electrostimulation on swimming performances
For EG, the swimming times declined significantly (P < 0.01) by 0.19 ± 0.14 s for the 25PB and by 0.38 ± 0.24 s for the 50FS. The stroke length increased significantly (P < 0.04) by 0.05 m·cycle⁻¹ but not the stroke rate. For CG, no statistical difference was measured for any of these variables (Table 2). For the whole group, the variations of the peak torques, measured in eccentric condition (-60 $°s^{-1}$), were related to the variations of the performances (r = 0.77; P < 0.01).

Table 2. Results of the pre- and post-raining performance times, stroke rate (SR), stroke length (SL) for the 7 electrostimulated (EG) and the 7 control (CG) swimmers.

	Pre-training				Post-training			
	25PB	50FS (s)	SR (c/min)	SL (m/c)	25PB	50FS (s)	SR (c/min)	SL (m/c)
EG	14.34	26.19	55.1	2.10	14.15 *	25.82 *	54.2	2.15 *
	(0.4)	(0.7)	(2.6)	(0.16)	(0.46)	(0.6)	(2.7)	(0.14)
CG	15.21	27.98	51.4	2.10	15.28	27.82	52.3	2.08
	(1.6)	(2.5)	(4.6)	(0.11)	(1.5)	(2.6)	(5.1)	(0.11)

* Significantly different from pre-training values.

4 Discussion

The main point of the present study was to indicate that electrostimulation of the latissimus dorsi enhanced muscular strength, performances and stroke length of a group of competitive swimmers compared to a control group.

4.1 Electrostimulation and muscle strength
In isometric conditions, the peak torque gain measured in the present study (+21%) was similar to those reported in the literature [1, 7]. In eccentric and concentric conditions at angular velocities higher than 180 $°s^{-1}$, the strength gain observed could be partly explained by a preferential adaptation of the fast twitch fibers, which could have been preferentially recruited during electrostimulation [8]. As a matter of fact, Thorstensson et al. [9] and Froese et al. [10] have reported that the percentage of fast twitch fibers was an important factor for the development of the maximal generated force. In such conditions, the composition of muscle fibers can even be predicted [11].

4.2 Electrostimulation and swimming performances
For the whole group of swimmers, the attempt to relate the arm strength to the performance was unsuccessful. This was probably due to the testing procedure used in the present study. As a matter of fact, the contribution of strength to the swimming performance has been clearly demonstrated by Johnson et al. [12]. These authors related different kinds of arm strength measurements to the performance on a 22.86-m swim. The highest correlation was found when the arm peak power was measured during swimming ($r = 0.87$ for 29 swimmers). Thus, to be significant, strength testing must be specific to the movement patterns used in swimming, explaining, therefore, the lack of a significant relationship between the peak torque and the performances found in the present study. Although muscle strength has been shown to be an important factor of success over short distances, the contribution of strength training to the performance has not been clearly explained. Costill et al. [3] and Sharp et al. [4] showed that after a strength training program, swimmers increased their mean power. The study of Tanaka et al. [5] differs. They showed that both swim training and combined swim and dry-land resistance training groups had significant but similar power gains as measured on a biokinetic swim bench. Moreover, no significant differences were found between the groups in any of the swim power and swimming performance tests. In the present study, the 7 swimmers of the electrostimulated group increased their peak torque on average by 10 to 24% and their performance by 1.3 and 1.4%. For the whole group, the variations of the peak torque were significantly related to the variations of the performances but only in eccentric condition (-60 $°s^{-1}$). This relation could be explained on the one hand by the fact that during eccentric contractions, fast twitch fibers were an important determinant for the strength development. On the other hand, by the fact that, in sprint, swimming performance require explosive force and fast twitch fibers. In the present study, the gains in performances of the electrostimulated swimmers were associated with an increase of the stroke length. Some studies [3, 13, 14] have demonstrated the importance of the stroke length in swimming. Hay and Guimaraes [15] have shown that the improvement of the velocity over the course of a season was almost exclusively due to corresponding improvements of stroke length. Craig et al. [14] have indicated that the decline of the velocity during a race was completely accounted for by the decreasing stroke length. The improvements in velocity between the 1976 and 1984 Olympic Games were attributable to increased stroke length and a decline in stroke rate in 16 out of 20 events. The authors suggested that stroke length variations were probably related to the ability to develop the force necessary to overcome resistance to forward movement [14].

In summary, this study indicates that an electrostimulation program of the latissimus dorsi increased the arm strength measured in isometric, eccentric and concentric conditions (over 180 °s⁻¹) and the swimming performances of a group of competitive swimmers compared to a control group. Thus, electrostimulation appears to be not only a rehabilitation means but also a possible useful means to develop specific arm strength in swimming.

References

1. Selkowitz, D.M. (1985) Improvement in isometric strength of the quadriceps femoris muscle after training with electrical stimulation. *Physical Therapy*, Vo. 65. pp. 186-196.
2. Rutherford, O. M. and Jones, D.A. (1986) The role of learning and coordination in strength training. *European Journal of Applied Physiology*, Vo. 55. pp. 100-105.
3. Costill, D., Sharp, R. and Troup, J. (1980) Muscle strength: contributions to sprint swimming. *Sports Medicine*, Vo 21. pp. 29-34.
4. Sharp, R.L., Troup, J. and Costil, D. L. (1982) Relationship between power and sprint freestyle swimmers. *Medicine and Science in Sports and Excercise*, Vo 14. pp. 53-56.
5. Tanaka, H., Costill, D. L., Thomas, R., Fink, W.J. and Widrick, J.J. (1993) Dry-land resistance training for competitive swimming. *Medicine and Science in Sports and Excercise*, 25. pp. 952-959.
6. Clarys, J.P. (1985) Hydrodynamics and electromyography: ergonomic aspects in aquatics. Applied Ergonomics, Vo. 16. pp. 11-24.
7. Hainaut K. and Duchateau, J. (1992) Neuromuscular electrical stimulation and voluntary exercice. *Sports Medicine*, Vo.14. pp. 100-113.
8. Enoka, R.M. (1988) Muscle strength and its development: new perspectives. *Sports Medicine*, Vo. 6. pp. 146-168.
9. Thorstensson, A., Grimby, G. and Karlsson, J. (1976) Force velocity relations and fiber composition in human knee extensor muscle. *Journal of Applied Physiology,* Vo. 40. pp. 12-16.
10. Froese, E.A. and. Houston, M.E. (1985) Torque-veloctiy characteristics and muscle fiber type in human vastus lateralis. *Journal of Applied Physiology*, Vo. 59. pp. 309-314.
11. Tihanyi, J., Apor, P. and Petrekanits, M. (1982) Force-velocity-power characteristics and fiber composition in human knee extensor muscles. *European Journal of Applied Physiology*, Vo. 48. pp. 331-343.
12. Johnson, R.E., Sharp, R.L. and Herick, C. E. (1993) Relationship of swimming power and dryland power to sprint freestyle performance: a multiple regression approach. *Journal of Swimming Research*, Vo. 9. pp. 10-14.
13. Chatard, J.C., Collomp, C., Maglischo, E. and Maglischo, C. (1990) Swimming skill and stroking characteristics of front crawl swimmers. *International Journal in Sports Medicine*, Vo. 11. pp. 156-161.
14. Craig, A.B., Skehan, P.L., Pawelczyk, J.A. and Boomer, W.L. (1985) Velocity, stroke rate, and distance per stroke during elite swimming competition. *Medicine and Science in Sports and Excercise*, Vo. 17. pp. 625-634.
15. Hay, J.G. and Guimaraes, A.C.S. (1983) A quantitative look at swimming biomechanics. *Swimming Technique*, Vo. 20. pp. 11-17.

Author index

Subject index

This index is compiled from the keywords assigned to the papers, edited and extended as appropriate. The page references are to the first page of the relevant paper.